KT-408-411

AN ILLUSTRATED COLOUR TEXT

OMY

AN ILLUSTRATED COLOUR TEXT

NEUROANATOMY

A. R. CROSSMAN PhD DSc

Professor of Anatomy,
School of Biological Sciences,
University of Manchester,
Manchester, UK

D. NEARY MD FRCP

Professor of Neurology,
University of Manchester,
Manchester, UK

Illustrated by
Raymond Evans and Denise Smith
Unit of Art in Medicine,
School of Biological Sciences,
University of Manchester,
Manchester, UK

CHURCHILL
LIVINGSTONE

EDINBURGH LONDON NEW YORK PHILADELPHIA SAN FRANCISCO SYDNEY
TORONTO 1998

CHURCHILL LIVINGSTONE
A Medical Division of Harcourt Brace and Company Limited

© Pearson Professional Limited 1995
© Harcourt Brace and Company Limited 1998

🐾 is a registered trademark of Harcourt Brace and
Company Limited

First published 1995
    Reprinted 1996
    Reprinted 1997
    Reprinted 1998

ISBN 0-443-04479-1

British Library of Cataloguing in Publication Data
A catalogue record for this book is available from the British Library.

Library of Congress Cataloging in Publication Data
A catalogue record for this book is available from the Library of
Congress.

Medical knowledge is constantly changing. As new information becomes available, changes in treatment, procedures, equipment and
the use of drugs become necessary. The editors / authors / contribu-
tors and the publishers have, as far as it is possible, taken care
to ensure that the information given in this text is accurate and up
to date. However, readers are strongly advised to confirm that
information, especially with regard to drug usage, complies with
the latest legislation and standards of practice.

**Cover image courtesy of
Philips Medical Systems.**

For Churchill Livingstone

Publisher: Timothy Horne
Project Editor: Jim Killgore
Designer: Sarah Cape
Pasteup Artist: Jim Farley
Production: Nancy Arnott / Kay Hunston
Sales Promotion: Duncan Jones

Produced by Addison Wesley Longman China Limited, Hong Kong.
GCC/04

Preface

This book has been written primarily for undergraduate medical students. At the same time, we have borne in mind students following other health science courses where a basic understanding of the nervous system and its major disorders is required, and also students of basic neuroscience, who are invariably intrigued and edified by discussion of the disorders which afflict the human nervous system.

The book has been prepared during a period of widespread debate on, and evolution in, the substance and style of medical education. There are several driving forces for change, one being the recognition that unreasonable and unnecessary demands are often being made of students in the sheer volume of information which they are required to assimilate. This has prompted students, educators and health professionals alike to question, across the whole curriculum, the depth of knowledge which is required by the newly-qualified doctor and the means by which it should be achieved. The General Medical Council has recommended the development of a system-based core curriculum and has emphasised the crucial importance of integration between basic science and clinical medicine. These proposals have been welcomed and amplified, with respect to the teaching of neurology, by the Association of British Neurologists.

No area of medical science lends itself better than neuroscience to such a system-based, integrated approach and this has been the principal philosophy guiding the preparation of this book. Neuroscience, with all its sub-specialities both basic and clinical, is an enormous field where the growth of knowledge through research is exponential. This creates a great challenge to the medical educator in selecting what should comprise the core curriculum. It also signifies the potential for future advances in the diagnosis, prevention and treatment of neurological disease, recognised by the designation of the 1990's as the 'Decade of the Brain'.

Neuroanatomy is the cornerstone upon which is built an understanding of the nervous system and its disorders. The aim of this book, therefore, is to provide a clear and concise account of the anatomy of the human nervous system in sufficient detail to understand its main functions and the common disorders by which it is affected. An important feature of the book is the integration of neuroanatomy with illustrative clinical material. This has been done in order to show how a knowledge of neuroanatomy can help in the understanding of clinical symptoms and also to emphasise those areas of neuroanatomy which are particularly relevant to human neurological disease. We have introduced clinical concepts in the most elementary way to give a broad outline of the aetiology of nervous disease and the link with clinical diagnostic methods. Clinical material has been integrated as closely as possible with the relevant neuroanatomy. Furthermore, the clinical text has been boxed so that it is readily identifiable and can be easily selected to review or pass over. Each chapter also contains boxed summaries. The purpose of these is to assist the reader in identifying key points and as an aid to revision.

Both neuroanatomy and clinical medicine are new to the student first entering Medical School. By studying the introductory chapter and the summaries of later, more detailed, chapters the student will gain an overview of the scope and extent of the subject of neuroanatomy and will be introduced to the basic concepts underlying the clinical diagnosis of neurological disease. For those unfamiliar with clinical terminology a glossary has been provided to explain the meaning of commonly-used expressions. As more detailed knowledge of neuroanatomy is gained, this will be enhanced and illuminated by reference to the selected clinical material which exemplifies the relevance of neuroanatomy to clinical neurology. Later, when students enter neurological training, they need to refresh in their minds the basic principles of neuroanatomy and link these to clinical diagnostic methods. At this time, the systematic study of patients with individual neurological diseases can be greatly enhanced by returning to the detailed anatomy of diseased structures.

Manchester
1995

A. R. Crossman
D. Neary

Acknowledgements

We wish to thank the numerous colleagues who have helped in so many ways to bring this book to publication. Within the School of Biological Sciences at Manchester University, our thanks go first and foremost to Raymond Evans and Denise Smith of the Unit of Art in Medicine for their patient, imaginative and skillful transformation of our elementary sketches and verbal descriptions into the many drawings which illustrate this book. We are also grateful to the director of the unit, Richard Neave, for his continual interest in the project and for making himself so readily available with help and advice.

The book contains many photographs of anatomical specimens and histological slides, the preparation of which has involved the technical skills of a number of individuals. We are grateful to anatomical dissecting room technicians John Davies and Mike Fish for helping to select the most suitable anatomical specimens for prosection and to John Hargreaves and Tony Bentley for their meticulous photography. We are also grateful to Frank Barnett and David Peggs for assistance with the preparation of stained brain slices and for their meticulous preparation of histological material. Although much of the manuscript was typed by the two-fingered, we are grateful to Ann Drozdowski for her intuitive and accurate transcription of many hand-written pages.

We are also indebted to Professor David Brooks, Consultant Neurologist at the MRC Cyclotron Unit, Hammersmith Hospital, London, for providing PET scans, to Dr. Alan Jackson, Consultant Radiologist in the Department of Radiology, Manchester Royal Infirmary, for providing MRI scans and to Dr. Paul Griffiths, Consultant Radiologist in the Department of Radiology, Newcastle General Hospital, Newcastle-upon-Tyne, for providing cerebral angiograms.

Of colleagues at Churchill Livingstone, we are especially grateful to publishing manager Timothy Horne and senior project editor Jim Killgore for their stimulating enthusiasm and calm patience and for steering us so professionally through the myriad stages of producing a book. We also wish to thank art director Ian Dick for his experienced guidance in the preparation of artwork and photographic material.

Manchester   A. R. C.
1995   D. N.

Contents

CHAPTER 1

Introduction to the nervous system

The human nervous system is the most complex and versatile achievement of the process of evolution. The nervous system of all animals functions to detect changes in the external and internal environment and to bring about appropriate responses in muscles, organs and glands. With ascent of the evolutionary scale there is, in addition, an increasing capacity for so-called 'higher functions' of the nervous system such as cognition, learning and memory and, ultimately, self-awareness, intellect and personality. The anatomical, physiological, biochemical and molecular bases of some aspects of neural function are fairly well understood whilst others occupy the professional lives of many thousands of researchers in both the basic and clinical sciences.

The nervous system is often damaged by inherited or developmental abnormalities, disease processes and by traumatic injury. The prevention, diagnosis and treatment of neurological disorders is, thus, of immense socio-economic importance. An understanding of neuroanatomy and its correlation with function and dysfunction may justifiably be regarded as a cornerstone for future advances in clinical neuroscience.

BASIC ORGANISATION OF THE NERVOUS SYSTEM

NEURONES AND NEUROGLIA

The basic structural and functional unit of the nervous system is the nerve cell or **neurone**, of which the human nervous system is estimated to contain about 10^{10}. The functions of the neurone are to receive and integrate incoming information from sensory receptors or other neurones and to transmit information to other neurones or effector organs. Its structure is highly specialised to fulfil these functions. Each neurone is a separate entity with a limiting cell membrane. Information is passed between neurones, therefore, at specialised regions called **synapses** where the membranes of adjacent cells are in close apposition (Fig. 1.1).

Although the diversity of neuronal types is wide, all share certain common characteristics. There is a single cell body from which a number of branching processes emerge. Most of these processes are receptive in function and are known as **dendrites**. They possess synaptic specialisations, sometimes many thousands of them, through which they receive information from other nerve cells with which they make contact. One of the processes leaving the cell body is called the **axon** or nerve fibre and this carries information away from the cell body. The axon may divide into several branches or **collaterals** by which means information can be distributed to a number of different destinations simultaneously. At the end of the axon, specialisations called **terminal boutons** occur, by which information is transferred to the dendrites of other neurones.

Information is coded within neurones by changes in electrical energy. The neurone at rest possesses an electrical potential (the **resting potential**) across its membrane of the order of 60–70 millivolts, the inside being negative with respect to the outside. When a neurone is stimulated or excited above a certain threshold there is a brief reversal of the polarity of its membrane potential, termed the **action potential**. Action potentials are propagated down the axon and invade the nerve terminals. Transmission of information between neurones

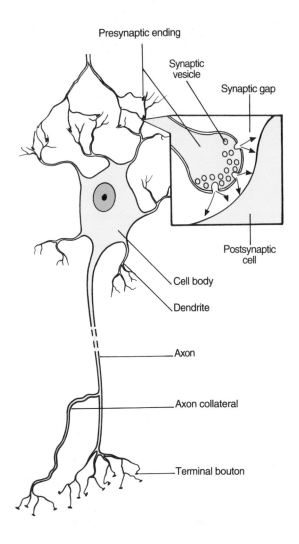

Fig. 1.1 **The basic structure of the neurone and the synapse.**

occurs, in the vast majority of instances, not by electrical but by chemical means. Invasion of nerve terminals by the action potential causes release of specific chemical agents, called **neurotransmitters,** which are stored in **synaptic vesicles** in the presynaptic ending. These diffuse across the narrow gap between pre- and post-synaptic membranes and bind to **receptors** on the postsynaptic cell, inducing changes in the membrane potential. The change may be either to depolarise the membrane and, thus, move towards the threshold for production of action potentials or it may be to hyperpolarise and, thus, stabilise the cell.

Neuroglial cells, or **glia**, constitute the other major cellular component of the nervous system, outnumbering neurones by an order of magnitude. Unlike neurones, neuroglia do not have a direct role in information processing but they fulfil a number of ancillary roles essential for the normal functioning of nerve cells. Three main types of neuroglial cells are recognised:

- **Oligodendroglia** form the **myelin sheath** that surrounds many neuronal axons, conferring increased rate of propagation of action potentials.

- **Astrocytes** are thought to form a selectively permeable barrier between the circulatory system and the neurones of the brain and spinal cord, the 'blood–brain barrier', which has a protective function.
- **Microglia** have a phagocytic role in the response to nervous system damage.

PERIPHERAL AND CENTRAL NERVOUS SYSTEMS

The nervous system is divided arbitrarily into the central nervous system (CNS) and the peripheral nervous system (PNS). The central nervous system consists of the brain and spinal cord, lying within the protection of the cranium and vertebral column, respectively. The peripheral nervous system consists of cranial and spinal nerves, together with their associated ramifications and ganglia, which link the CNS with sensory receptors and with effector organs (muscles and glands).

The nervous system is also considered to consist of two principal functional divisions: the somatic and autonomic nervous systems. Both of these have components in the CNS and PNS. The autonomic nervous system controls visceral functions and homeostatic mechanisms. It is considered more fully in Chapter 14.

AFFERENT NEURONES, EFFERENT NEURONES AND INTERNEURONES

Nerve cells which carry information from peripheral receptors to the central nervous system are referred to as **afferent neurones**. If the information which they carry ultimately reaches a conscious level they are also called **sensory neurones. Efferent neurones** carry impulses away from the central nervous system. Those that innervate skeletal muscle and cause movement are also referred to as **motor neurones**. The vast majority of neurones, however, reside entirely within the central nervous system. They are sometimes referred to as **interneurones** or **internuncial neurones**. The terms 'afferent' and 'efferent' are also commonly used to denote projections to and from structures within the CNS even though the projections are entirely contained within the brain and spinal cord. One may refer to the projections to and from the cerebral cortex, for example, as cortical afferents and efferents, respectively.

GREY AND WHITE MATTER, NUCLEI AND TRACTS

The central nervous system is a highly heterogeneous structure in terms of the distribution of nerve cell bodies and their processes. Some regions are relatively enriched in nerve cell bodies (e.g. the central portion of the spinal cord, the surface of the cerebral hemisphere) and are referred to as **grey matter**. Other regions contain mostly nerve processes (usually axons). These are often myelinated (ensheathed in myelin) which confers a whitish colouration — hence the term **white matter**.

Nerve cell bodies with similar anatomical connections and functions (e.g. the motor neurones innervating a group of related muscles) tend to be located together in groups called **nuclei**. Similarly, nerve processes sharing common connections and functions tend to follow the same course, running in pathways or **tracts**.

DECUSSATION OF SENSORY AND MOTOR PATHWAYS

It is a general principle of the organisation of the central nervous system that pathways conveying sensory information to a conscious level (the cerebral hemisphere) cross over, or **decussate**, from one side of the CNS to the other. The same is true of descending pathways from the cerebral hemisphere, which control movement. Thus, in general, each cerebral hemisphere perceives sensations from, and controls the movements of, the contralateral side of the body.

Basic organisation of the nervous system

- The basic structural and functional unit of the nervous system is the nerve cell, or neurone.
- Information is passed between neurones by chemical transmission at synapses.
- A neurone receives information primarily through its dendrites.
- Action potentials are carried away from the cell body by the axon and influence other neurones by release of neurotransmitter from presynaptic terminals.
- By acting upon receptors in the postsynaptic membrane the neurotransmitter causes either depolarisation or hyperpolarisation of the postsynaptic cell.
- Neuroglial cells are more numerous than nerve cells but are not directly involved in information processing. They are important for normal neural function because of their ancillary roles.
- Oligodendrocytes form the myelin sheath which surrounds axons and increases their rate of conduction.
- Astrocytes may form the blood–brain barrier.
- Microglia have a phagocytic function when the nervous system is damaged.
- The nervous system is divided into the central nervous system (CNS), which consist of the brain and spinal cord, and the peripheral nervous system (PNS).
- Individual neurones may be defined as either afferent or efferent with respect to the CNS, or as interneurones.
- Within the CNS, areas rich in either nerve cell bodies or fibres constitute grey and white matter, respectively.
- Clusters of cell bodies with similar functions are known as nuclei.
- Tracts of nerve fibres link distant regions.
- Generally, ascending sensory and descending motor pathways in the CNS decussate along their course, so that each side of the brain is functionally associated with the contralateral half of the body.

BASIC DEVELOPMENT AND ORGANISATION OF THE CENTRAL NERVOUS SYSTEM

The nervous system is derived from the embryonic ectoderm. During the third week of embryonic development, the dorsal midline ectoderm undergoes thickening to form the **neural plate** (Fig. 1.2). The lateral margins of the neural plate become elevated forming

Fig. 1.2 **The formation of the neural tube from the embryonic ectoderm**.

neural folds on either side of a longitudinal, midline depression, the **neural groove**. The neural folds then become apposed and fuse together, thus sealing the neural groove and creating the **neural tube**. Some cells from the apices of the neural folds become separated to form groups lying dorsolateral to the neural tube. These are known as the **neural crests**. The formation of the neural tube is complete by about the middle of the fourth week of embryonic development.

Enormous growth, distortion and cellular differentiation occur during the subsequent transformation of the neural tube into the adult central nervous system. This is maximal in the rostral part, which develops into the brain, the caudal portion becoming the spinal cord. The central cavity within the neural tube becomes the central canal of the spinal cord and the ventricles of the brain. The neural crests form the sensory ganglia of spinal and cranial nerves, and also the autonomic ganglia.

As development continues, a longitudinal groove, the **sulcus limitans**, appears on the inner surface of the lateral walls of the embryonic spinal cord and caudal part of the brain (Fig. 1.3A). The dorsal and ventral cell groupings thus delineated are referred to as the **alar plate** and the **basal plate**, respectively. Nerve cells which develop within the alar plate have predominantly sensory functions, whilst those in the basal plate are predominantly motor. Further development also brings about the differentiation of grey and white matter. The grey matter is located centrally around the central canal, with white matter forming an outer coat.

BASIC ORGANISATION OF THE SPINAL CORD

The spinal cord is relatively undifferentiated in comparison to the brain. Thus, the basic principles of organisation, established early in embryonic development, can be readily identified even in the adult human cord (Fig. 1.3B).

The spinal cord is basically cylindrical in shape and contains at its centre a vestigial **central canal**. The separation of cell bodies from nerve fibres gives a characteristic 'H' or 'butterfly' shape to the central core of grey matter which surrounds the central canal. Four extensions of the central grey protrude dorsolaterally and ventrolaterally towards the surface. These are known as **dorsal horns** and **ventral horns**, respectively. The dorsal horn is the site of termination of many afferent neurones, conveying impulses from sensory receptors throughout the body, and is the site of origin of ascending pathways carrying sensory impulses to the brain. The ventral horn contains motor neurones which innervate skeletal muscle.

The spinal cord receives information from, and controls, the trunk and limbs. This is achieved through bilaterally paired **spinal nerves** which join the cord at intervals along its length. Near to the cord the spinal nerves divide into **dorsal** and **ventral roots** which

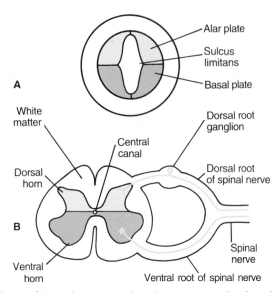

Fig. 1.3 **Schematic representation of transverse section through (A) developing neural tube and (B) adult spinal cord**.

attach to the cord near to the tips of the dorsal and ventral horns, respectively. The dorsal roots carry afferent fibres, whose cell bodies are located in **dorsal root ganglia**. The ventral roots carry efferent fibres whose cell bodies of origin lie within the spinal grey matter.

The periphery of the cord consists of white matter which contains longitudinally running nerve fibres. These are organised into a series of ascending tracts, which carry information from the trunk and limbs to the brain, and descending tracts, by which the brain controls the activities of the spinal cord.

Basic organisation of the spinal cord

- The spinal cord consists of a central core of grey matter and an outer layer of white matter.
- Within the white matter run ascending and descending nerve fibre tracts which link the spinal cord with the brain.
- The spinal cord bears paired spinal nerves by which it receives fibres from and sends fibres to the periphery.
- Near the cord, spinal nerves form dorsal and ventral roots: dorsal roots carry afferent fibres, whose cell bodies lie in dorsal root ganglia; ventral roots carry efferent fibres.

BASIC ORGANISATION OF THE BRAIN
Embryonic development and structure

During embryonic development the rostral portion of the neural tube undergoes massive differentiation and growth to form the brain (Fig. 1.4). By the fifth week, three primary brain vesicles can be identified: the **prosencephalon** (forebrain), **mesencephalon** (midbrain) and **rhombencephalon** (hindbrain). By the seventh week further differentiation distinguishes five secondary brain vesicles, due to the division of the prosencephalon into **telencephalon** and **diencephalon** and division of the rhombencephalon into **metencephalon** and **myelencephalon**. The neuraxis does not remain straight but is bent by a **midbrain** or **cephalic flexure**, occurring at the junction of midbrain and forebrain, and a **cervical flexure** between the brain and spinal cord.

Some of the names of the embryological subdivisions of the brain are commonly used for descriptive purposes and it is, therefore, useful to know the parts of the mature brain into which they subsequently develop (Table 1.1). Of the three basic divisions of the brain, the prosencephalon or forebrain is by far the largest. It is also referred to as the **cerebrum**. Within the cere-

brum, the telencephalon undergoes the greatest further development and gives rise to the two **cerebral hemispheres**. These consist of an outer layer of grey matter (the **cerebral cortex**) and an inner mass of white matter, within which various groups of nuclei lie buried (the largest being the **corpus striatum**). The diencephalon consists largely of the **thalamus**, which contains numerous cell groupings and is intimately connected with the cerebral cortex. The mesencephalon, or midbrain, is relatively undifferentiated (it still retains a central tube-like cavity surrounded by grey matter). The metencephalon develops into the **pons** and overlying **cerebellum**, whilst the myelencephalon forms the **medulla oblongata** (medulla). By convention, the medulla, pons and midbrain are collectively referred to as the **brain stem** (Fig. 1.5).

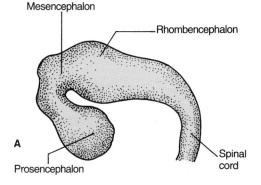

Table 1.1 **Embryonic development of the brain**

Primary brain vesicles	Secondary brain vesicles	Derivatives in mature brain
Prosencephalon (forebrain)	Telencephalon	Cerebral hemisphere
	Diencephalon	Thalamus
Mesencephalon (midbrain)	Mesencephalon	Midbrain
Rhombencephalon (hindbrain)	Metencephalon	Pons, cerebellum
	Myelencephalon	Medulla oblongata

Fig. 1.4 **The early development of the brain showing the (A) primary and (B) secondary brain vesicles**. (Modified with permission from Barr ML, Kiernan JA 1993, *The Human Nervous System*, 6th edn. J.B. Lippincott, Philadelphia.)

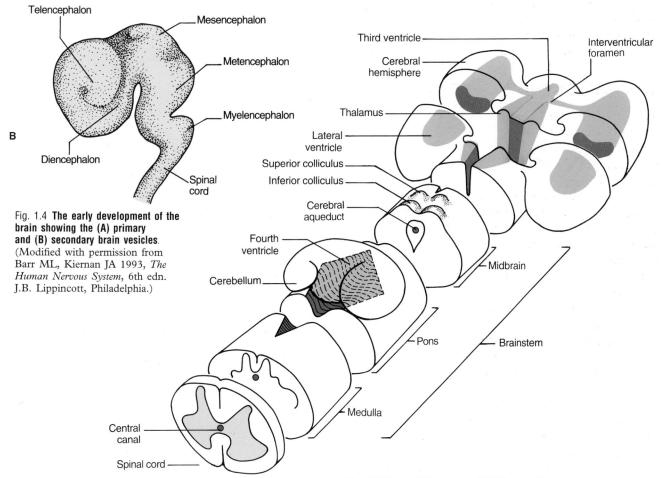

Fig. 1.5 **Some of the major subdivisions and landmarks of the brain**.

As the brain develops, its central cavity also undergoes considerable changes in size and shape forming a system of chambers or **ventricles**, which contain **cerebrospinal fluid** (CSF) (Fig 1.5).

Parallels have sometimes been drawn between the embryological development of the brain and the major changes which the brain has undergone during ascent of the phylogenetic, or evolutionary, scale from simple to more complex animals. Whilst certainly an over-simplification, this concept does have the advantage of introducing some of the principal parts of the brain, and their relationships to one another, in a graphic and memorable way (Fig. 1.5).

The simplest of chordate animals (e.g. amphioxus), from which the vertebrates evolved, possesses a dorsal tubular nerve cord which is reminiscent of the neural tube of the developing mammalian embryo. During phylogeny the rostral end of the tubular nervous sys-

Fig. 1.6 **Photographs of the brain**.
(**A**) Lateral aspect; (**B**) median sagittal section;
(**C**) dorsal aspect; (**D**) ventral aspect.

tem has undergone enormous modification and change so that the adult human brain bears little obvious similarity to its evolutionary ancestors.

Regional specialisation has been an important theme in the evolution of the brain and this is especially obvious in relation to the senses and in movement control. Long ago in phylogeny, centres devoted to these functions developed as expansions or outgrowths from the dorsal aspect of the simple tubular brain (Fig. 1.5). In form they consisted of an outer cortex of nerve cell bodies with an underlying core of nerve fibres. Bilaterally paired centres developed in relation to the senses of smell, vision and hearing, and a symmetrical, midline centre developed in association with vestibular func-

tion and the maintenance of equilibrium. Each of these centres underwent subsequent evolutionary change, but this was most evident in the rostral, 'olfactory', part of the brain which developed into the massive cerebral hemispheres (Figs 1.6 and 1.7). During this process of prosencephalisation the cerebral hemispheres came to take on an executive role in many areas of brain function. Thus, for example, the highest level for perception and correlation of all sensory modalities eventually became localised in the cortical surface of the cerebral hemispheres, as did the highest level for motor control. This is reflected by the fact that only a small proportion of the adult human cerebral hemisphere remains directly related to olfactory function.

Fig. 1.7 **Principal subdivisions and some important landmarks In the mature brain**.
(**A**) Median sagittal section; (**B**) ventral aspect.
Cranial nerves are indicated in yellow.

The process of prosencephalisation has meant that the other centres became progressively subservient to the cerebral hemispheres. For example, those for vision and hearing underwent relatively little development and fulfil largely automatic, reflex functions in the human brain. They may still be identified, however, as four small swellings on the dorsal surface of the midbrain: the **corpora quadrigemina** or **superior** and **inferior colliculi** (Figs 1.5, 1.7). The motor centre near the caudal end of the brain developed into the cerebellum (Figs 1.5, 1.6 and 1.7) which retains a very important role in the coordination of movement.

Ventricular system

The highly simplified plan of the basic brain described above is a useful one on which to consider the general disposition of the ventricular system (Fig. 1.5; see also Figs 1.7 and 1.8). As the central canal of the spinal cord ascends into the brain stem it moves progressively in a dorsal direction, eventually opening out to form a shallow, rhomboid-shaped depression on the dorsal surface of the medulla and pons (the hindbrain portion of the brain stem) beneath the cerebellum. This is the **fourth ventricle**.

At the rostral border of the pons the walls of the fourth ventricle converge forming once again a narrow tube, the **cerebral aqueduct** (Figs 1.5, 1.7 and 1.8). The cerebral aqueduct dives into the substance of the brain stem running the length of the midbrain, beneath the inferior and superior colliculi. At the junction of midbrain and forebrain the aqueduct opens into the **third ventricle** (Figs 1.5, 1.7 and 1.8), a slit-like chamber, narrow from side-to-side but extensive in

dorsoventral and rostrocaudal dimensions. The lateral walls of the third ventricle are formed by the diencephalon, the major part of which constitutes the thalamus. Near the rostral end of the third ventricle a small aperture, the **interventricular foramen** or **foramen of Monro** (Figs 1.5, 1.7 and 1.8), communicates with an extensive chamber, the **lateral ventricle** (Figs 1.5 and 1.8), within each cerebral hemisphere.

Brain stem

When the brain is viewed externally the massive cerebral hemispheres obscure many other structures, but a median sagittal section (Figs 1.6 and 1.7) reveals most of the main features of the basic brain. The brain stem can be clearly seen on both a median sagittal section and ventral view (Figs 1.6 and 1.7) of the brain. The brain stem consists of the medulla oblongata, pons and midbrain, each of which can be readily delineated.

The brain stem constitutes only a small proportion of the entire brain but it is crucially important. Through it pass nerve fibre tracts linking the brain and spinal cord, which are essential for the receipt of sensory information from, and control of, the limbs. It also contains the sites of origin and termination of many of the **cranial nerves** through which the brain innervates the head region. Moreover, within the brain stem lie centres controlling the vital functions such as respiration and the cardiovascular system.

The medulla oblongata is continuous caudally with the spinal cord and extends rostrally as far as the pons. This can be clearly seen on ventral or sagittal views since the ventral part of the pons forms a prominent bulge on the surface of the brain stem. In sagittal

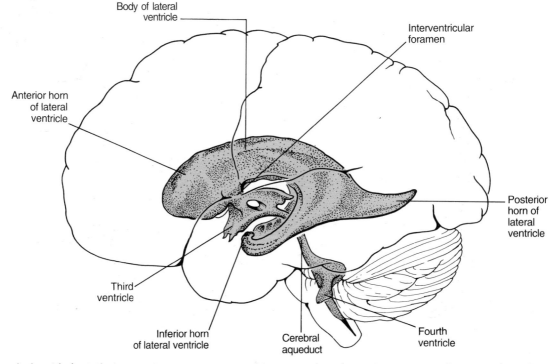

Fig. 1.8 **The cerebral ventricular system**.

section (Figs 1.6 and 1.7), the lumen of the fourth ventricle can be seen between the pons and medulla ventrally and the cerebellum dorsally, into which its tent-shaped roof extends. The cerebellum is attached to the brain stem by a large mass of nerve fibres which lie lateral to the fourth ventricle on either side. It is split nominally into three parts: the **inferior, middle** and **superior cerebellar peduncles**.

These carry nerve fibres between the medulla, pons and midbrain, respectively, and the cerebellum. The largest cerebellar peduncle is the middle and it is the only one readily seen without further dissection (Fig. 1.7B). The cerebellum consists of an outer layer of grey matter, the cerebellar cortex, surrounding a central core of white matter. The cortical surface is highly convoluted to form a regular pattern of narrow, parallel folds or **folia**. The cerebellar white matter consists of nerve fibres running to and from the cortex. It has a characteristic branching, tree-like arrangement in section (Figs 1.6 and 8.6), as its ramifications reach towards the surface.

Rostral to the pons is located the relatively small midbrain. On its dorsal surface can be seen the rounded eminences of the superior and inferior colliculi, beneath which runs the cerebral aqueduct (Figs 1.5, 1.6, 1.7).

Diencephalon and cerebral hemispheres

Rostral to the brain stem lies the forebrain, consisting of the diencephalon and cerebral hemispheres. The diencephalon and cerebral hemisphere on each side of the brain are to a large extent physically separate from their counterparts on the other side, although important cross-connections do exist, as will be discussed shortly. The two sides of the diencephalon are separated by the lumen of the third ventricle, whose lateral walls they constitute.

The diencephalon consists of four main subdivisions in a dorsoventral direction: the **epithalamus, thalamus, subthalamus,** and **hypothalamus**. The epithalamus is small and its most notable component on a sagittal section is the **pineal gland**, which lies in the midline, immediately rostral to the superior colliculi of the midbrain (Fig. 1.7A). The thalamus is by far the largest part of the diencephalon and it forms much of the lateral wall of the third ventricle. Little of the subthalamus can be seen and its structure and function are considered elsewhere (Ch. 11). The hypothalamus forms the lower part of the walls, and also the floor, of the third ventricle. It is a highly complex and important region because of its involvement in many systems, most notable being the autonomic nervous system (Ch. 14), the limbic system and the neuro-endocrine system (Ch. 13). From the ventral aspect of the hypothalamus in the midline arises the **infundibulum** or pituitary stalk to which is attached, in life, the **pituitary gland** (Fig. 1.7).

The cerebral hemisphere is by far the largest part of the brain. Like the cerebellum, it consists of an outer layer, or cortex, of grey matter and an inner mass of white matter (Figs 1.9, 1.10). In addition, buried within

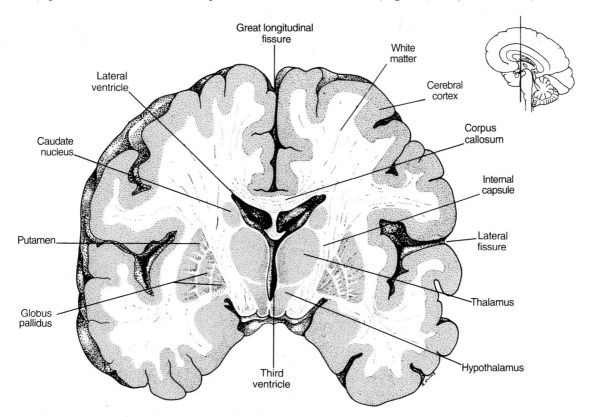

Fig. 1.9 **Drawing of a coronal section through the cerebral hemisphere at the level of the interventricular foramen.**

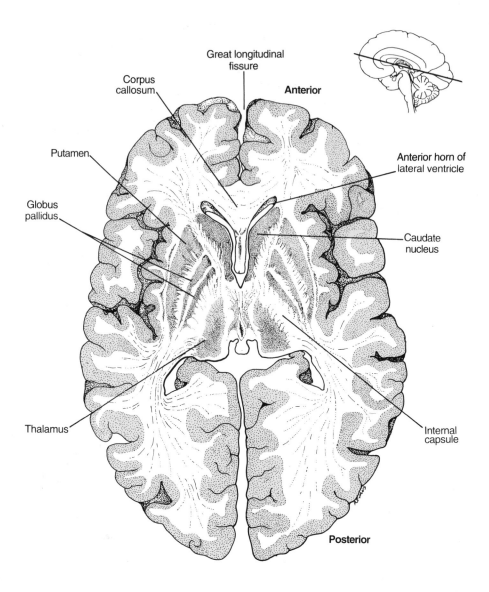

Fig. 1.10 **Drawing of an approximately horizontal section through the cerebral hemisphere**.

the white matter lie several large masses of cell bodies collectively referred to as the basal ganglia (Figs 1.9 and 1.10). The two cerebral hemispheres are separated by a deep midline cleft, the **great longitudinal fissure** (Fig. 1.9), which in life accommodates the **falx cerebri**, a sheet of dura mater reflected from the internal surface of the cranium. In the depths of the fissure lies the **corpus callosum** (Figs 1.7A, 1.9), an enormous sheet of transversely running nerve fibres (commissural fibres) which link corresponding areas of the two cerebral cortices.

The cerebral cortex is highly convoluted. This has the effect of maximising the cortical surface area, which is over one square metre for each hemisphere. The convolutions are called **gyri** (singular: gyrus) and the furrows between them are **sulci** (singular: sulcus). Some gyri and sulci are consistently located from brain to brain and mark the location of important functional areas.

On the lateral surface of the hemisphere a deep cleft, the **lateral fissure** (Figs 1.9, 1.11), is an important landmark. This, together with certain sulci, constitutes boundaries which divide the hemisphere into four lobes (Figs 1.11 and 1.12). The lobes bear the names of the bones of the skull beneath which they lie.

The most anterior part of the cerebral hemisphere is called the **frontal lobe**, the most anterior convexity of which is the frontal pole. The posterior boundary of the frontal lobe is the **central sulcus** which can readily be identified as a single, continuous furrow running over the entire lateral surface of the hemisphere, from the great longitudinal fissure to the lateral fissure. Posterior to the central sulcus lies the **parietal lobe**, which is separated from the **temporal lobe** below by the lateral fissure. The tip of the temporal lobe is called the temporal pole. The posterior part of the hemisphere is the **occipital lobe**, ending in the occipital pole. The boundaries between parietal and temporal lobes and

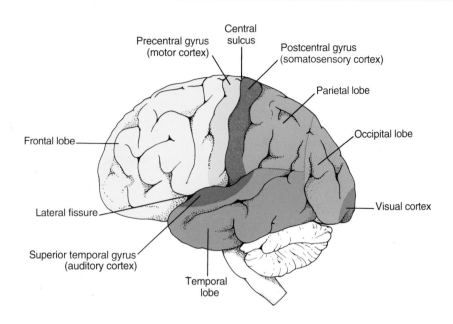

Fig. 1.11 **Lateral aspect of the brain**.
The figure illustrates some of the principal gyri, sulci and functional areas.

the occipital lobe are indistinct on the lateral surface of the hemisphere since they do not correspond to any particular sulci, but on the medial surface parietal and occipital lobes are separated by a deep **parieto-occipital sulcus** (Fig. 1.12).

The functions of the cerebral cortex are described in more detail in Chapter 10. It will be useful at the outset, however, to identify four important functional areas of cortex, one in each lobe (Figs 1.11 and 1.12).

- In the frontal lobe, the gyrus immediately in front of the central sulcus is referred to anatomically as the **precentral gyrus**. Functionally, this contains the **primary motor cortex**, which is the highest level in the brain for the control of movement. Here, in each hemisphere, the opposite half of the body is represented in a highly precise fashion.
- In the parietal lobe, facing the primary motor cortex across the central sulcus, lies the **postcentral gyrus** or **primary somatosensory cortex**. This is the site of termination of pathways carrying the modalities of touch, pressure, pain and temperature from the opposite half of the body and it is the region where they are consciously perceived. The special senses have their highest level of representation in other areas.
- The **visual cortex** is located in the occipital lobe, mostly on the medial aspect of the hemisphere in the gyri above and below the horizontally orientated **calcarine sulcus**.
- In the temporal lobe lies the **auditory cortex**. It is localised to the **superior temporal gyrus** which lies beneath, and parallel to, the lateral fissure.

During development, the cerebral hemisphere takes on a C-shaped configuration due to the forward migra-

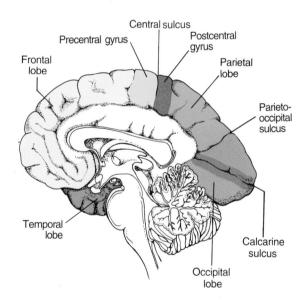

Fig. 1.12 **Sagittal section of the brain**.
The figure illustrates some of the principal gyri, sulci and functional areas.

tion of the temporal lobe, such that the temporal pole lies adjacent to the frontal lobe and separated from it by the lateral fissure. The lateral ventricle within the hemisphere thus also is basically C-shaped with 'horns' extending into the frontal, occipital and temporal lobes (Fig. 1.8).

The basic structure of the cerebral hemisphere is an outer mantle of grey matter, the cerebral cortex, be-

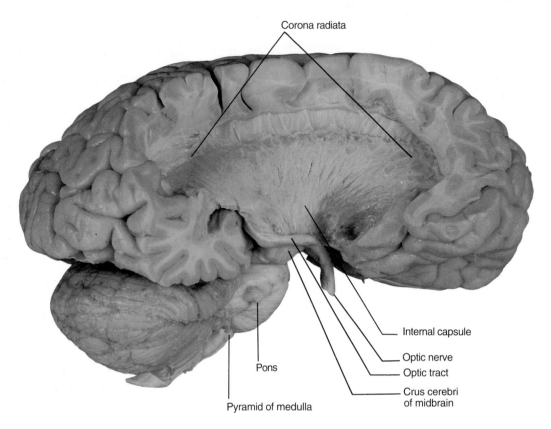

Corona radiata

Internal capsule

Optic nerve

Optic tract

Crus cerebri
of midbrain

Pons

Pyramid of medulla

Fig. 1.13 **Dissection of the brain from the lateral aspect**.
The figure illustrates the corona radiata and the internal capsule.

neath which lies a large and complex mass of white matter consisting of nerve fibres running to and from the cortex (Figs 1.9, 1.10 and 1.13).

Cortical afferent and efferent fibres which pass between the cerebral cortex and subcortical structures, such as the corpus striatum, thalamus, brain stem and spinal cord are arranged in a characteristic radiating pattern, the **corona radiata**, which reaches out to the convolutions of the cortical surface (Fig. 1.13). Deeper inside the hemisphere the fibres are concentrated into a dense sheet of white matter, known as the **internal capsule** (Figs 1.9, 1.10 and 1.13).

Deep inside the hemisphere, both medial and lateral to the internal capsule, lie additional masses of grey matter. The largest of these is the **corpus striatum**, which consists of the **caudate nucleus**, **putamen** and **globus pallidus** (Figs 1.9 and 1.10). The caudate nucleus lies in the wall of the lateral ventricle throughout its extent and, like the ventricle, it is therefore C-shaped.

Basic organisation of the brain

- The brain is conventionally divided into hindbrain, midbrain and forebrain.
- The hindbrain is further subdivided into the medulla oblongata, pons and cerebellum.
- The medulla, pons and midbrain constitute the brain stem.
- The forebrain consists of the diencephalon (thalamus and hypothalamus) and the cerebral hemisphere.
- Within the cerebral hemisphere lie several large nuclei called the basal ganglia or corpus striatum.
- The brain contains a system of cavities or ventricles containing cerebrospinal fluid which is produced by the choroid plexus.
- The brain possesses 12 pairs of cranial nerves which carry afferent and efferent fibres.
- The two cerebral hemispheres are linked by the fibres of the corpus callosum.
- The surface of the cerebral hemisphere consists of cortical grey matter, which is folded to form gyri and sulci.
- Beneath the surface lie the dense fibre masses of the corona radiata and the internal capsule.
The surface of the hemisphere is divided into 4 lobes:
- The frontal lobe contains the primary motor and premotor cortices.
- The parietal lobe contains the primary somatosensory cortex.
- The temporal lobe contains the primary auditory cortex.
- The occipital lobe contains the primary visual cortex.

BASIC CLINICAL DIAGNOSTIC PRINCIPLES

A knowledge of neuroanatomy is a prerequisite for the clinical diagnosis of disorders of the nervous system. The process of diagnosis proceeds by history taking, the neurological examination and finally by confirmatory investigations (Fig. 1.14). History taking provides clues to the aetiology or cause of disease, whereas the clinical examination pinpoints the site of the lesion (Fig. 1.15). A pathological lesion acting at a specific locality within the neuromuscular axis forms a recognisable syndrome, investigation of which leads to establishing the aetiology or diagnosis.

AETIOLOGY OF NEUROLOGICAL DISEASE

Disorders of the neuromuscular system are of four major types (Fig. 1.16).

Extrinsic disorders are due to acute trauma or chronic mechanical compression (Fig. 1.17) and they have priority of investigation, which is directed to neurosurgical management and the operative relief of the source of compression.

Fig. 1.14 **The process of clinical diagnosis**.

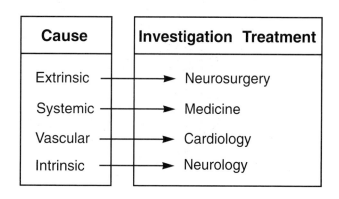

Cause	Investigation Treatment
Extrinsic	Neurosurgery
Systemic	Medicine
Vascular	Cardiology
Intrinsic	Neurology

Fig. 1.16 **The four major categories of disorders of the neuromuscular system**.

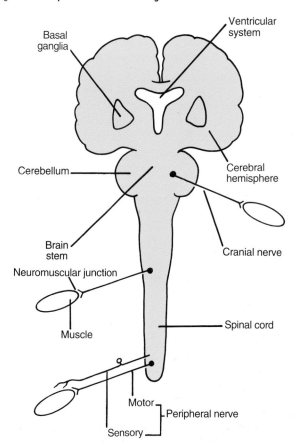

Fig. 1.15 **The central and peripheral nervous systems and possible sites of pathological lesion**.

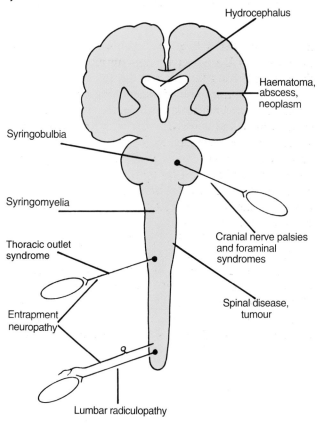

Fig. 1.17 **Extrinsic disorders of the nervous system**.

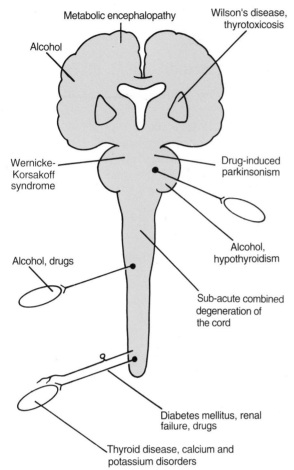

Fig. 1.18 **Systemic disorders of the neuromuscular system**.

Vascular disorders damage the circulation to the nervous system:

- occlusion of the vessels (**thrombosis**)
- restricting the blood and oxygen supply (**infarction**)
- bleeding into the nervous tissues (**haemorrhage**).

The rapid development of a vascular lesion is called a **stroke**. Congenital swellings of arteries (**aneurysms**) or tumours of blood vessels (**angiomas**) can compress cranial nerves and the brain itself. Investigations are directed to discovering abnormalities of the blood, the functions of the heart, the state of the great vessels in the chest and neck and the arteries and veins of the brain, spinal cord, nerves and muscles. Management of this group of disorders is often cardiological.

Intrinsic disorders are primary disorders of the nervous system (Fig. 1.19). Many nervous disorders are under genetic influences. **Inborn errors of metabolism** lead to mental subnormality and disability in children and are usually due to deficiency of specific enzymes. In youth and in adults, **system degenerations** occur leading to loss of specific tissues (atrophy) with preservation of other systems. The degenerations are chronic disorders (Fig. 1.20). **Paroxysmal disorders** consist of episodic loss of consciousness (epilepsy), excessive sleep (narcolepsy) and headache (migraine). **Neoplasia** refers to excessive uncontrolled growth of tissues forming a benign or malignant tumour. Primary neoplasms arise in the neuromuscular tissues themselves (Fig. 1.21); secondary neoplasms spread in the circulation from other primary organ sites (e.g. lung or breast). Rarely, tumours at distant sites damage the nervous system by humoural or immune mechanisms and the resulting disorders are termed non-metastatic, or paraneoplastic, syndromes (Fig. 1.22). **Inflammation** of neuromuscular tissue may be due to infection caused by microorganisms (Fig. 1.23) or to immune reactions in the absence of obvious infection (Fig. 1.24).

Systemic disorders are primarily of organs other than the nervous system but disrupt neuromuscular function by abnormal metabolism (Fig. 1.18). Investigations are directed to unearthing systemic disease for management and control by the appropriate speciality within internal medicine.

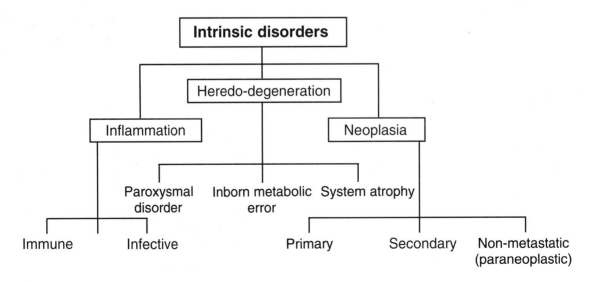

Fig. 1.19 **Intrinsic disorders of the nervous system**.

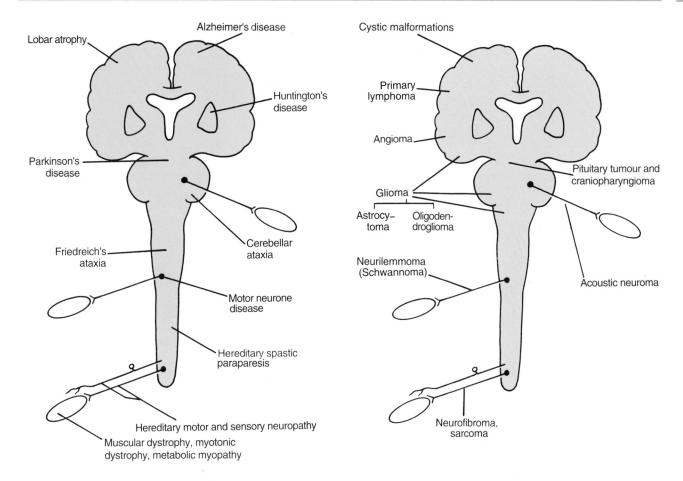

Fig. 1.20 **Degenerative disorders of the neuromuscular system.**

Fig. 1.21 **Neoplasia of the nervous system.**

Fig. 1.22 **Non-metastatic (paraneoplastic) syndromes of the neuromuscular system.**

Fig. 1.23 **Infections of the neuromuscular system.**

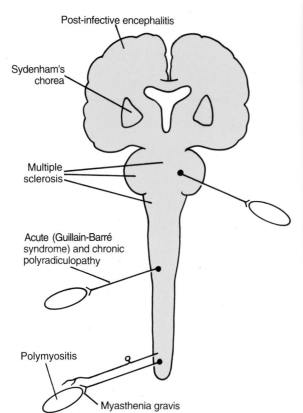

Post-infective encephalitis

Sydenham's chorea

Multiple sclerosis

Acute (Guillain-Barré syndrome) and chronic polyradiculopathy

Polymyositis

Myasthenia gravis

Fig. 1.24 **Immune disorders of the neuromuscular system.**

Fig. 1.25 **T1-weighted magnetic resonance image of the brain.** (Courtesy of Dr. A. Jackson, Department of Diagnostic Radiology, University of Manchester)

SITE OF THE LESION AND CLINICAL SYNDROMES

Whatever the cause (aetiology) of the lesion or lesions, their site in the neuromuscular system leads to characteristic syndromes revealed by examination of the cranial nerves, the motor system, the reflexes, sensation and finally coordination. These systems are depicted diagrammatically (see Fig. 1.26) so that the syndromes can be illustrated pictorially in a way that links neuroanatomy with clinical signs and underlines the necessary knowledge of each in the diagnostic process. In order to forge such links the major routes of the sensory and motor pathways, the significance of lesions of the 'upper motor neurone' and 'lower motor neurone' (p. 54) and the general functions of the cerebellum and basal ganglia must be appreciated.

INVESTIGATION OF NEUROMUSCULAR DISEASE

The clinical definition of a particular syndrome permits the choice of appropriate investigations to confirm the diagnosis. The major focus of investigations involves:

- cerebrospinal fluid (CSF) analysis
- neuroradiology
- neurophysiology
- neuropathology (biopsy).

Lumbar puncture (see p. 41) enables the measurement of CSF pressure and the collection of CSF for bacteriological, biochemical, serological and cytological analyses. These may reveal the presence of blood (subarachnoid haemorrhage), infection, immune disease such as multiple sclerosis or the presence of tumour cells.

Neuroradiology encompasses straight X-ray imaging of the skull and vertebral column, structural imaging of the brain and spinal cord (**computed tomography (CT)** and **magnetic resonance imaging** (MRI, Fig. 1.25) and functional imaging of cerebral blood flow and metabolism (**single photon emission tomography** (SPECT) and **positron emission tomography** (PET)).

In contrast radiology an opaque medium is injected into the arteries or veins (**angiography**) to delineate the blood vessels or into the spinal canal (**myelography**) to outline the spinal cord and nerve roots.

Neurophysiology addresses the electrical activity of the central nervous system by **electroencephalography** (EEG) and the detection and measurement of **evoked responses** to visual, auditory and somatosensory stimuli. **Central magnetic stimulation** to the brain enables measurement of the motor conduction time to the spinal cord and limb muscles. In the peripheral nervous system, measures of motor and sensory **nerve conduction velocity** and evoked **sensory action potentials** are combined with measurement of individual muscle responses to voluntary and electrically-evoked contraction (**electromyography**).

The **biopsy** of nerve, muscle and brain tissue sheds light on the pathophysiological process (e.g. axonal degeneration, demyelination, muscular degeneration) and on the aetiology (e.g. inflammation, neoplasia).

Clinical detail

Throughout the text, simplified outlines of the major anatomical–clinical syndromes are presented diagrammatically following the conventional neurological examination of cranial nerves, motor function, reflexes, sensation and coordination and mental state described in textbooks of clinical methods (Fig. 1.26).

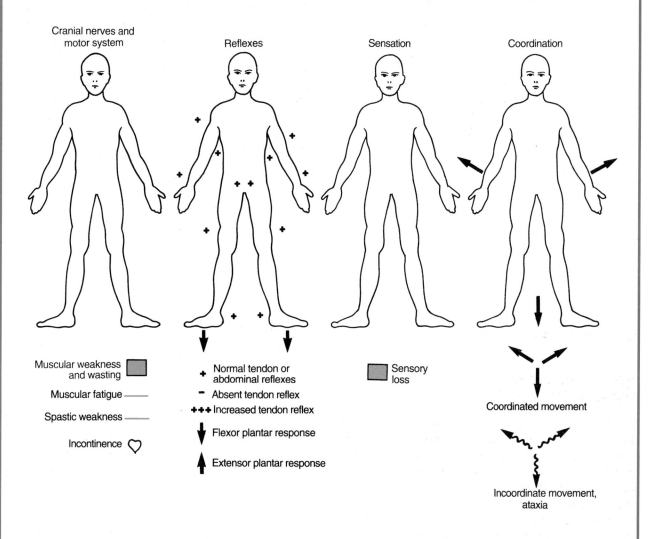

Fig. 1.26 Prototypical figure for illustration of major syndromes of the neuromuscular system.

Basic clinical diagnostic principles

- History taking, clinical examination and investigations lead to the diagnosis of the cause (aetiology) of disease.
- The site of the lesion(s) determines the clinical syndrome revealed by the neurological examination.
- Disorders of the nervous system can be classified as extrinsic, systemic, vascular or intrinsic.
- Intrinsic disorders consist of system degenerations (atrophy), inborn errors of metabolism, paroxysmal disorders, neoplasms, infections and immune disorders.

Cells of the nervous system

The principal functional unit of the nervous system is the nerve cell or neurone. These cells are highly specialised for the encoding, conduction and transmission of information. Present in even larger numbers are neuroglial cells, or glia. These do not take part directly in information processing but are, nonetheless, crucial for normal neural function. Other cells are also present in the nervous system, such as those forming the walls of blood vessels but, unlike neurones and neuroglia, these are not unique to the nervous system.

THE NEURONE

SIZE AND STRUCTURE

The main structural features, common to all neurones, have been described briefly in Chapter 1. There are, however, numerous variations of the basic plan. The size of the cell body varies considerably depending upon location and function. For example, some interneurones in the CNS have cell bodies as small as 5 microns in diameter, whilst the cell bodies of motor neurones innervating striated muscle may exceed 100 microns. The size of the cell body is usually correlated with the length of the axon. Thus, a small interneurone will have a short axon, perhaps only a fraction of a milli-metre in length. A large motor neurone will possess a long axon (e.g. those passing from the spinal cord to the muscles of the foot have axons about 1 metre long).

The **dendritic arborisation** of neurones also shows great variation in the number, size and density of branches, which reflect the organisation of afferent inputs to the cell. This is illustrated by considering the dendritic arborisations of, for example, a pyramidal cell in the cerebral cortex and Purkinje cell in the cerebellar cortex (Fig. 2.1).

Fig. 2.1 **A pyramidal cell from the cerebral cortex (A) (× 100) and a Purkinje cell from the cerebellar cortex (B) showing the diversity of dendritic arborisations (× 90)** Golgi–Cox stain.

Like most other cells, neurones possess a nucleus. This is usually located in the centre of the cell body and contains the neurone's chromosomal DNA. The rest of the intracellular space is occupied by cytoplasm which contains numerous organelles and inclusions (Fig. 2.2). Many of these are common to cells other than neurones but some have particular prominence or significance in neurones. Numerous microscopic clumps of **Nissl substance** or granules can usually be seen in nerve cell bodies stained with basophilic dyes. Nissl substance consists of rough endoplasmic reticulum and associated ribosomes. The ribosomes contain RNA (which accounts for the basophilic staining properties) and are the sites of protein synthesis. Nerve cells are highly metabolically active and, therefore, the Nissl substance is often very prominent (Fig. 2.3).

Neurones contain a complex meshwork of structural protein strands called **neurofilaments**, which are assembled into larger **neurofibrils** (Fig. 2.2). They also possess a system of **microtubules** which are involved in the transport of materials throughout the cell. Transport of materials occurs both away from, and towards, the cell body (anterograde and retrograde

Fig. 2.3 **A spinal motor neurone cell body**.
Cresyl violet (a basophilic dye) stain shows prominent Nissl substance (× 600).

transport, respectively). This phenomenon is exploited in certain neuroanatomical tracing techniques.

Some neurones contain pigment granules. **Neuro-melanin** is a brownish-black pigment produced as a by-product of the synthesis of catecholamines. Neuromelanin occurs most prominently in certain cell groups known to utilise catecholamines as their neurotransmitter, notably the substantia nigra, pars compacta, of the midbrain and the locus coeruleus of the pons. **Lipofuscin** is a yellowish-brown pigment which accumulates in certain neurones with age.

Each nerve cell in the nervous system is a separate physical entity. In order for information processing to occur in networks of neurones, therefore, information has to pass between neurones. This occurs at synapses. The basic structure of the synapse has been outlined in Chapter 1 (p. 2). The most common location for synapse formation is between the terminal axonal arborisation of one neurone and the dendrite of another (**axodendritic** synapse). Other locations are also possible and they give axosomatic, axoaxonal and dendrodendritic synapses. Neurotransmission occurs by release of specific chemical agents from the presynaptic element which act upon receptors on the postsynaptic membrane.

NEUROTRANSMITTERS

Neurotransmitter chemicals are stored in vesicles within the presynaptic ending. A single neurone is thought to release the same transmitter at all its synapses and all neurones of a particular type, in terms of origin, termination and function, utilise the same transmitter. Numerous transmitter substances have been identified at various sites in the nervous system. It has long been known that **acetylcholine** (ACh) is the transmitter between motor neurones and striated muscle. It is also the transmitter at autonomic ganglia and is released by postganglionic parasympathetic neurones. Some amino

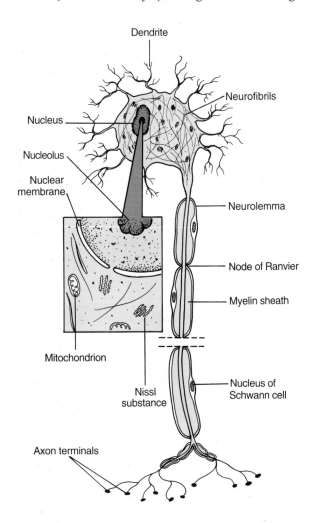

Fig. 2.2 **A typical neurone**.
The diagram illustrates the principal structural features, some intracellular organelles and the myelin sheath.

acids act as neurotransmitters, most notably **glutamic acid** and **gamma aminobutyric acid** (GABA) which are widespread throughout the CNS. Several mono-amines are important transmitters. **Noradrenaline** is released by postganglionic sympathetic neurones peripherally as well as at many sites within the CNS. **Dopamine** and **serotonin** (5-hydroxytryptamine, 5-HT) also act as transmitters in the brain and spinal cord.

The effect of the neurotransmitter must be terminated once it has acted upon the postsynaptic membrane. This is achieved either by enzymic destruction or re-uptake of the transmitter into nerve endings and glia. For example, the effect of acetylcholine at neurone/neurone synapses and the neuromuscular junction (Fig. 3.3, p. 25) is terminated by the action of the enzyme acetycholinesterase. On the other hand, monoamines are usually inactivated by a re-uptake mechanism.

A large number of peptides are also known, or thought, to be stored and released at synapses. These include **enkephalin, substance P, cholecystokinin, somatostatin, dynorphin** and many others. These peptides are often found co-localised in the same neurones as amino acid or amine transmitters. It is believed that the peptides modulate the release and postsynaptic effects of other transmitters and they are, therefore, often referred to as **neuromodulators**.

Fig. 2.4 **An astrocyte showing a process forming a perivascular end-foot on a blood capillary.**
Cajal's gold chloride stain (× 180).

Astrocytes

Astrocytes possess numerous processes. Some of these form so-called 'perivascular end-feet' upon the walls of blood capillaries (Fig. 2.4). Astrocytes are probably involved in the exchange of chemicals between the circulatory system and nervous tissue. It has been suggested that they may constitute the 'blood–brain barrier' which restricts the access of circulating chemicals to the brain and spinal cord.

Oligodendroglia

Oligodendroglia possess few processes. Their main role is production of the myelin sheath which surrounds many axons in the CNS. **Schwann cells** perform this function in the peripheral nervous system. Myelination increases the rate of conduction of axons. The myelin sheath consists of numerous concentric layers of oligodendrocyte or Schwann cell membrane (Fig. 2.5). Each glial cell produces the myelin sheath over only a short

---

The neurone

- The neurone is the principal functional unit of the nervous system, specialised for the receipt, processing and transmission of information.
- Great variability exists in the size and shape of nerve cell bodies, their dendritic arborisations and axons, which reflects their functional specialisation.
- Nerve cells contain a number of organelles and inclusions. Amongst these are: Nissl substance, neurofilaments and microtubules and pigment granules.
- A large number of neurotransmitter substances are known which mediate transmission between neurones. These include primarily acetylcholine, various amino acids (GABA, glutamate) and catecholamines (noradrenaline and dopamine).
- Peptide neuromodulators are co-localised in many neurones.

NEUROGLIA

Neuroglia are not directly involved in information processing but they are important for normal functioning of the nervous system. Various types of neuroglial cells are recognised, principally astrocytes, oligodendroglia (oligodendrocytes) and microglia.

Neuronal and glial disorders

Once development has been acheived, individual neurones no longer replicate, but undergo continual repair to maintain their integrity. Hence, they are prone to **neurodegenerative diseases** which in childhood and youth are often genetically determined and in the elderly are sporadic. Glia, unlike neurones, are capable of replication and they are, therefore, susceptible to neoplasia. Consequently, most brain tumours are gliomas and not tumours of neurones themselves. According to the cell of origin they may become either **oligodendrogliomas** or **astrocytomas**. Microglia form part of the immune system and may proliferate to become cerebral **lymphomas**.

Axon

Nucleus of Schwann cell

Fig. 2.5 **Transverse section through a myelinated axon**.
The diagram illustrates the structure of the myelin sheath.

segment of axon (up to about 1 mm). A long axon is, therefore, enveloped by the membranes of many glial cells. Adjacent segments of myelin, derived from different glial cells, are separated by a small gap, the **node of Ranvier** (Fig. 2.2). Ionic fluxes across the axonal membrane, which mediate generation of the action potential, occur only at the nodes of Ranvier where the axon is exposed. Between nodes, where the axon is insulated by myelin, depolarisation spreads by passive means (electrotonus). This means of propagation is known as **saltatory conduction** (Latin: saltare, to jump), since the action potential may be thought of as 'jumping' from node to node. It is considerably faster than conduction in unmyelinated axons.

Multiple sclerosis

The myelin sheath of neuronal axons can be the seat of inflammatory diseases. In Europe and North America the commonest immune disorder of the CNS is multiple sclerosis, which leads to episodes of demyelination and remyelination of axons, corresponding to relapses and remission of neurological symptoms and signs. Since the disorder is chiefly of axons, not cell bodies, magnetic resonance brain imaging can detect abnormal signals from demyelinating foci in the cerebral white matter.

Microglia

Microglia are small cells with few processes. Microglia increase in number at sites of damage in the central nervous system and have a phagocytic role, similar to macrophages elsewhere. The ependyma consists of epithelial cells which line the ventricles and cover the choroid plexus.

Neuroglia

- Neuroglia are important for normal neural function because of their ancillary roles.
- Astrocytes possess long processes which form perivascular end-feet around blood capillaries. They are involved in the transfer of materials between the vascular system and neural tissue.
- Oligodendroglia give rise to the myelin sheath surrounding axons in the CNS. Schwann cells form myelin in the peripheral nervous system.
- Microglia have a phagocytic role in injury to the nervous system.

Peripheral nervous system

The peripheral nervous system consists of nerve endings, peripheral nerve trunks, plexuses and ganglia which link the central nervous system with other parts of the body. Many of the neurones in the peripheral nervous system are, therefore, either afferent or efferent with respect to the CNS.

- *Nerve endings* include sensory receptors which detect changes in the internal and external environments and effector endings which control the contraction of muscle and the activity of secretory glands.
- *Peripheral nerves* consist of spinal and cranial nerves and their branches and the numerous named nerves to which these give rise.
- *Plexuses*, e.g. the brachial plexus and lumbosacral plexus, are structures in which fibres within spinal and cranial nerves are redistributed, without synapse, to form other peripheral nerves.
- *Ganglia* are the locations of peripheral nerve cell bodies, e.g. dorsal root ganglia and autonomic ganglia.

MUSCLE

All behaviour depends on our ability to control the activity of the skeletal muscles which maintain posture and permit movement. Such control is subserved by a rich innervation of muscle with both motor and sensory neurones. Individual muscle cells run parallel to the main axis of the muscle and may be regarded as falling into two main functional groups, namely **extrafusal** and **intrafusal**.

Extrafusal muscle cells are by far the more numerous, constitute the bulk of the muscle and confer its contractile strength. These muscle cells are innervated by alpha motor neurones whose cell bodies lie in the ventral horn of the spinal cord or the motor cranial nerve nuclei of the brain stem. An individual alpha motor neurone typically branches within the muscle to innervate a number of muscle cells simultaneously, the combination of neurone and muscle fibres which it innervates being known as a **motor unit**. Motor units are small in those muscles with which delicate, precise movements can be made, such as the muscles of the hand and the extraocular muscles. Motor neurone axons end upon muscle cells in synaptic specialisations called **neuromuscular junctions** or **motor end-plates**.

Intrafusal muscle fibres are highly specialised cells which act as stretch and tension receptors. They occur in groups known as **muscle spindles**. There are two types of intrafusal muscle fibre, referred to as **nuclear bag** and **nuclear chain** fibres. They bear two types of sensory ending, known as **annulospiral** and **flower-spray endings**, which become activated when the muscle in which they lie is stretched. Intrafusal muscle cells also bear motor endings which are innervated by gamma motor neurones. These regulate the sensitivity of the sensory endings to applied stretch. Muscle spindles and their functional importance in motor control are considered in more detail in Chapter 5.

NERVE ENDINGS

Nerve endings may be classified as either sensory or effector. Sensory endings respond to mechanical, thermal or chemical stimulation, the nerve fibre to which they belong conducting action potentials to the CNS. Effector endings contact muscle or secretory cells and, under control from the CNS, produce movement or influence secretion.

SENSORY ENDINGS

The sensory systems or modalities, are broadly divided

Myopathies

Myopathy is characterised by weakness and wasting (of facial, bulbar and proximal limb muscles) with preservation of tendon reflexes and sensation (Fig. 3.1); also refer to Chapter 1, Figure 1.26.

Polymyositis is an immune disorder of muscle causing a painful or painless myopathy. When it occurs in the elderly there is often a primary neoplasm elsewhere (non-metastatic syndrome). In children the skin is also inflamed, causing a rash. This is referred to as dermatomyositis.

Duchenne muscular dystrophy is an inherited degenerative disorder of male children (x-linked inheritance). After 2–3 years of age the child develops progressive weakness of the arms and legs with muscular contractures. He is wheel-chair bound by the age of 10 years and dies in youth.

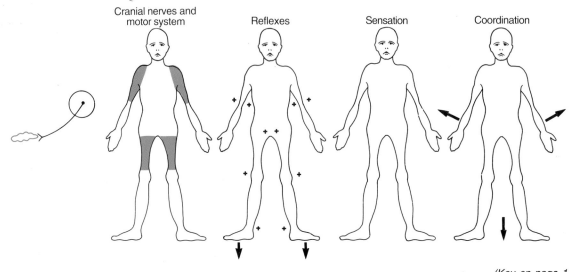

Fig. 3.1 **Myopathy**.

(Key on page 17)

---

into the general and the special senses. The special senses of vision, hearing, balance, olfaction and taste are considered elsewhere. General sensory endings are described as:

- **Exteroceptors**. These occur superficially in the skin and respond to nociceptive (painful) stimuli, temperature, touch and pressure.
- **Interoceptors**. These occur in viscera.
- **Proprioceptors**. These occur in muscles, joints and tendons and provide awareness of posture and movement (kinaesthesia).

Structurally, sensory nerve endings may be either unencapsulated or encapsulated (Fig. 3.2). Unencapsulated or **free nerve endings** consist of the terminal branches of sensory nerve fibres, lying freely in the innervated tissue. They appear to mediate thermal and painful sensations. Encapsulated nerve endings are surrounded by a structural specialisation of non-neural tissue, the combination of nerve and its encapsulation often being referred to as a corpuscle. For example, **Meissner's corpuscles** occur in the skin and are particularly numerous in the dermal papillae of the fingertips. They respond with great sensitivity to touch and are thought to be responsible for fine, or discriminative, touch. **Pacinian corpuscles** also occur in skin and in deep tissues, e.g. surrounding joints and in mesentery. They respond to mechanical distortion. Within skeletal muscles, intrafusal muscle fibres, which in small groups constitute **muscle spindles**, respond to muscle stretch. They are particularly abundant in muscles capable of fine, skilled movements. They are important in the control of muscle tone, movement and kinaesthesia and are described more fully in Chapter 5 (p. 44). Golgi tendon organs occur in tendons and respond to tension.

EFFECTOR ENDINGS

Effector endings occur in association with muscle and secretory cells. The endings resemble synapses which occur between neurones. Transmission is by chemical means, depolarisation of the endings causing release of a neurotransmitter which acts upon the target cell membrane. The motor end-plate or neuromuscular junction is a specialised ending in striated muscle. Motor axons divide to supply a widely variable number of muscle fibres (Fig. 3.3). A single axon and the muscle fibres which it innervates, constitute a motor unit. The neurotransmitter released at the neuromuscular junction in striated muscle is acetylcholine.

Fig. 3.3 **Motor end-plates in striated muscle**.
(**A**) Ranvier's gold chloride stain showing efferent nerve fibres and neuromuscular junctions (× 600). (**B**) Acetylcholine esterase stain. The neurotransmitter at the neuromuscular junction is acetylcholine. The action of the transmitter is terminated by the enzyme acetylcholine esterase. This stain shows the specific localisation of the enzyme at the neuromuscular junction (× 500).

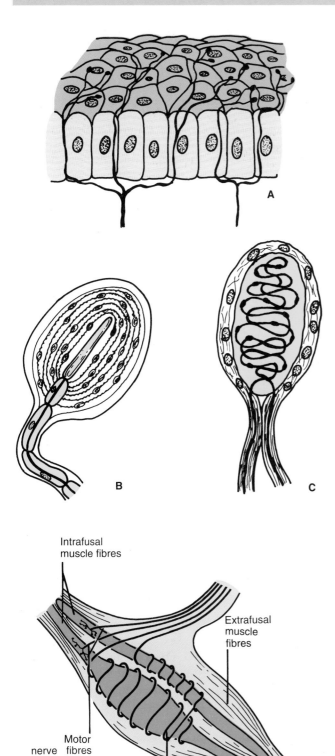

Fig. 3.2 **Sensory nerve endings**.
(**A**) Free nerve endings; (**B**) Pacinian corpuscle; (**C**) Meissner's corpuscle; (**D**) Muscle spindle.

Nerve endings

- The peripheral nervous system consists of nerve endings, peripheral nerves, plexuses and ganglia.
- Nerve endings are broadly classified as sensory or effector.
- Sensory endings are functionally subdivided into exteroceptors, interoceptors and proprioceptors.
- Structurally, they may consist of unencapsulated, or free, nerve endings or encapsulated endings (such as Meissner's and Pacinian corpuscles).
- Skeletal muscles contain intrafusal muscle fibres which form muscle spindles.
- Effector endings are either neuromuscular endings or endings in association with secretory cells.

Myasthenia gravis is an immune disorder and is the commonest disorder of the peripheral neuromuscular junction. It causes weakness and fatigue of cranial muscles (e.g. extraocular, facial and bulbar muscles) and limb (especially proximal) muscles. This occurs without muscular wasting, changes in reflexes or sensation (Fig. 3.4); also refer to Ch. 1, Fig. 1.26).

Treatment with anticholinesterase drugs potentiates neuromuscular transmission, with relief of symptoms. Intravenous edrophonium (Tensilon) is a diagnostic test for the disease and produces rapid, but brief, return of muscular power. The **Eaton–Lambert syndrome** causes similar fatigue, but is a non-metastatic syndrome and does not respond to anticholinesterases.

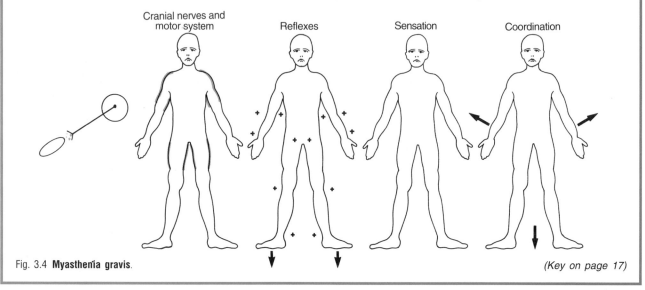

Fig. 3.4 **Myasthenia gravis**.   *(Key on page 17)*

PERIPHERAL NERVES

The term peripheral nerve encompasses all the nerve trunks and branches which lie outside the central nervous system. They are the principal route through which the brain and spinal cord communicate with the rest of the body. A typical peripheral nerve consists of numerous nerve fibres which may be either afferent or efferent with respect to the CNS.

Some peripheral nerve fibres are myelinated; others are unmyelinated. Within peripheral nerves, the nerve fibres are arranged in bundles and surrounded by sheaths of connective tissue (Fig. 3.5). Between individual fibres is a delicate connective tissue known as **endoneurium**. Bundles of fibres are surrounded by **perineurium** and the whole nerve is ensheathed by a tough coat known as **epineurium**. This configuration conveys strength and support to the nerve. The cranial and spinal meninges are continuous with the connective tissue sheaths of spinal and cranial nerves. Thus, the dura mater is continuous with the epineurium, whilst the arachnoid and pia are continuous with the perineurium and endoneurium.

DEGENERATION AND REGENERATION

When a peripheral nerve fibre is transected or otherwise seriously damaged, the portion distal to the

Fig. 3.5 **The structure of a peripheral nerve**.

Peripheral sensorimotor neuropathies

Peripheral sensorimotor neuropathies are characterised by muscular weakness and wasting (especially of distal muscles), distal areflexia and a 'glove and stocking' distribution of sensory loss (Fig. 3.6). Peripheral neuropathies may be due to systemic disease, vascular disease, heredodegenerative disorders, infection, immune disorders and non-metastatic syndromes. In general there are two pathological types. **Demyelinating neuropathies** predominantly damage Schwann cells and myelin sheaths. **Axonal neuropathies** primarily cause axonal degeneration. Recovery from neuropathy requires remyelination and regeneration of axons.

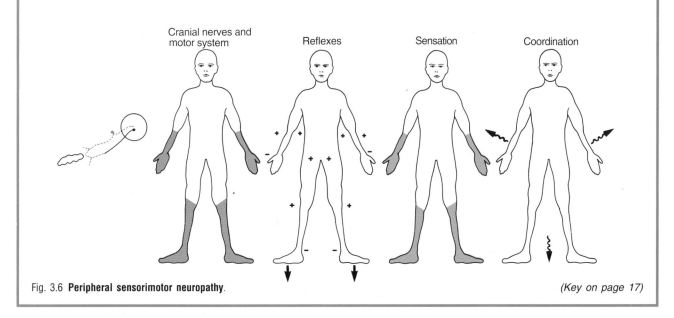

Fig. 3.6 **Peripheral sensorimotor neuropathy**. *(Key on page 17)*

transection dies and undergoes degeneration. This is known as **anterograde** or **Wallerian degeneration**. The proximal portion of the neurone, which remains attached to the cell body, may, however, survive and eventually undergo recovery or **regeneration**. The further from the cell body that transection occurs, the more likely it is that the cell will survive. Initially, it too usually shows degenerative changes, known as **retrograde degeneration**. This is characterised by dispersal and loss of staining of Nissl substance within the cell body (chromatolysis), swelling of the cell body and movement of the normally central nucleus to a peripheral location. If the cell recovers, the distal end of the surviving nerve fibre undergoes sprouting. If the two ends of the peripheral nerve are physically aligned, the new regenerating fibres may enter the endoneurial tubes which have lost their nerve fibres. Continued growth of the new fibres, at a rate of 1–2 mm a day, may eventually lead to reinnervation of the original structure and recovery of function. Many factors influence the degree to which successful reinnervation and functional recovery take place.

The degenerative processes which follow nerve cell injury are essentially similar in the central nervous system. Sprouting of surviving neurones also occurs in the CNS, but the reestablishment of previous connections does not, unfortunately, take place to any significant extent.

DISTRIBUTION OF SPINAL AND PERIPHERAL NERVES

At the roots of the upper and lower limbs are located the brachial plexus (Fig. 3.7) and lumbosacral plexus, respectively. Here, the nerve fibres present in spinal nerves become redistributed to form named peripheral nerves which then run distally to their targets. The distribution of peripheral nerves is, therefore, different from that of spinal nerves.

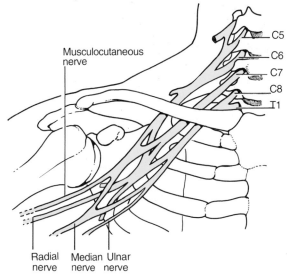

Fig. 3.7 **The brachial plexus**.

Brachial plexus lesions

In motor cycle accidents, trauma to the shoulder and neck may cause **avulsion of the brachial plexus**, causing immediate weakness and loss of feeling in one upper limb. Later, the arm wastes and becomes painful.

A tumour of the apex of the lung may infiltrate the lower part of the brachial plexus, producing severe pain in the arm, weakness and wasting of the hand and sensory loss on the inner aspect of the forearm and hand (**Pancoast's syndrome**).

Each spinal nerve carries the sensory innervation for a part of the body surface. The area of skin which is supplied by a particular spinal nerve is known as a **dermatome**. Dermatome maps are given in Figure 3.8. These are only approximate, since in reality the cutaneous territories of adjacent spinal nerves overlap considerably. The cutaneous distribution of important peripheral nerves is also illustrated in Figure 3.8.

The group of skeletal muscles innervated by a particular spinal nerve are collectively known as a **myotome**. These muscles are usually functionally related and are responsible for particular patterns of movement. The segmental spinal nerve values of some important movements are shown in Figure 3.9.

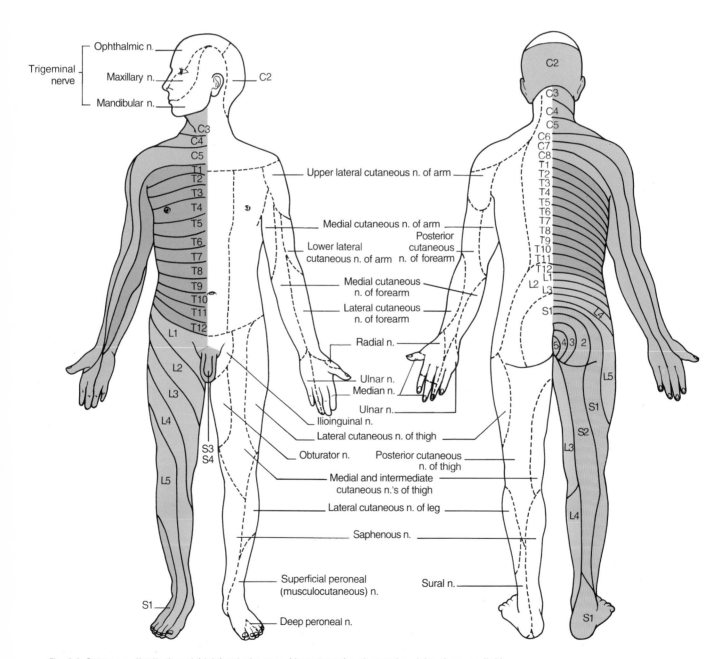

Fig. 3.8 **Cutaneous distribution of (right) spinal nerves (dermatomes) and named peripheral nerves (left)**. The cutaneous distribution of the three divisions of the trigeminal nerve is also illustrated.

Fig. 3.9 **The segmental innervation of limb movements**.
(**A**) Upper limb; (**B**) lower limb.

Compression and entrapment neuropathies

Peripheral nerves are vulnerable to extrinsic compression (e.g. excessive pressure on a recumbent limb) and to chronic entrapment by normal or diseased anatomical structures adjacent to them. The commonest examples are **radial nerve** compression in the spiral groove of the humerus, chronic entrapment of the **ulnar nerve** at the elbow and **median nerve** at the wrist (carpal tunnel syndrome) in the upper limb. Entrapment of the **lateral cutaneous nerve of the thigh** and compression of the **common peroneal nerve** at the head of the fibula, occur in the lower limb (Fig. 3.10).

Ulnar nerve

Sensory	Motor
	Small muscles of the hand except abductor pollicis brevis
	Ulnar half of flexor digitorum profundus
	Flexor carpi ulnaris

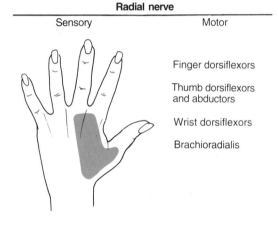

Median nerve

Sensory	Motor
	Abductor pollicis brevis

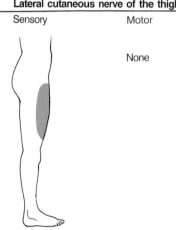

Radial nerve

Sensory	Motor
	Finger dorsiflexors
	Thumb dorsiflexors and abductors
	Wrist dorsiflexors
	Brachioradialis

Lateral cutaneous nerve of the thigh

Sensory	Motor
	None

Common peroneal nerve

Sensory	Motor
	Toe dorsiflexors
	Foot dorsiflexors
	Foot evertors

Fig. 3.10 **Sensory and motor deficits in peripheral nerve lesions**.

Peripheral nerves

- Peripheral nerves consist of variable numbers of bundles, or fascicles, of nerve fibres.
- Fibres are ensheathed in three connective tissue coverings: endoneurium, perineurium and epineurium.
- The endoneurial tubes within which individual axons lie are important for successful regeneration and reinnervation by peripheral nerves following nerve injury.
- Many nerve fibres in cranial and spinal nerves become rearranged as they course peripherally, by passage through nerve plexuses.
- The area of skin supplied by a spinal nerve is called a dermatome.
- The group of muscles innervated by a spinal nerve is called a myotome.

Coverings of the central nervous system

The central nervous system is supported and protected by bone and membranous coverings. The brain is located within the cranial cavity of the skull and the spinal cord lies in the vertebral, or spinal, canal within the vertebral column, or spine. Within their bony coverings the brain and spinal cord are invested by three concentric membranous envelopes. The outermost membrane is the **dura mater**, the middle layer is the **arachnoid mater** and the innermost layer is the **pia mater**. The vertebral column and spinal meninges are described in Chapter 5 and, thus, only the skull and cranial meninges are considered here.

SKULL

The brain lies on the floor of the cranial cavity which, together with the bones of the cranial vault, provides support and protection from physical injury. The floor of the cranial cavity consists of three **fossae**. Each of these accommodates particular parts of the brain and possesses **foramina** through which cranial nerves and blood vessels enter and leave the cranial cavity (Fig. 4.1).

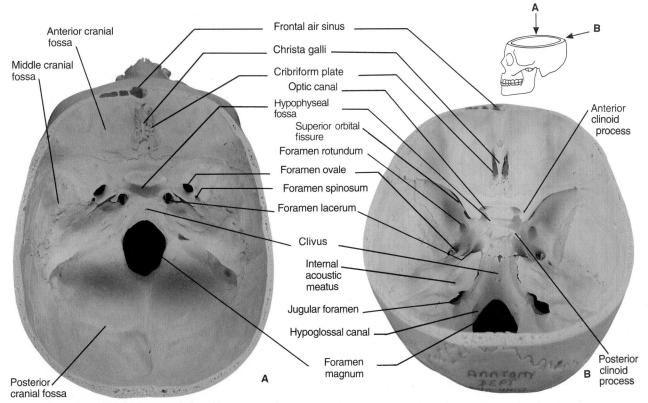

Fig. 4.1 **Floor of the skull showing the three cranial fossae and principal foramina.**

Anterior cranial fossa

The anterior cranial fossa is formed by the frontal, ethmoid and sphenoid bones. It contains the frontal lobes of the brain. The greater part of the floor of the anterior cranial fossa consists of the frontal bone and also forms the roof of the orbit. The part of the frontal bone which forms the anterior wall of the fossa contains the **frontal air sinus**. In the midline of the floor of the anterior cranial fossa is the ethmoid bone. In the midline a sharp ridge, the crista galli, provides attachment for the falx cerebri. In a depression on either side of the crista galli lie the **cribriform plates** of the ethmoid. These accommodate the **olfactory bulbs**. The bone of the cribriform plate is peppered with small perforations, through which the fascicles of the olfactory nerve enter the cranial cavity from the nasal cavity, to attach to the olfactory bulb.

Middle cranial fossa

The middle cranial fossa is formed by the sphenoid and temporal bones. In the midline the body of the sphenoid forms a deep depression, the **hypophyseal fossa**, en-compassed by four spurs of bone, the anterior and posterior clinoid processes. In the hypophyseal fossa lies the **hypophysis**, or **pituitary gland**. Lateral to the body of the sphenoid, the rest of the middle cranial fossa contains the temporal lobes of the cerebral hemisphere. The middle cranial fossa contains numerous points of entry and exit from the cranial cavity for cranial nerves and blood vessels.

- The **optic canal** is located medial to the anterior clinoid process and communicates with the orbit. Through it pass the optic (II) nerve and the ophthalmic artery (a branch of the internal carotid artery).
- The **superior orbital fissure** lies between the greater and lesser wings of the sphenoid bone and also communicates with the orbit. It carries the oculomotor (III), trochlear (IV) and abducens (VI) nerves and the ophthalmic division of the trigeminal (V) nerve.

Raised intracranial pressure

A **space-occupying lesion** is an expanding focal lesion such as a tumour, haematoma or abscess. Since the cranial cavity is closed and unyielding, the brain is distorted and displaced downwards, towards the foramen magnum, as the intracranial pressure rises. The patient complains of headache, vomiting, blurring of vision and drowsiness. The optic discs are swollen (**papilloedema**), signs of brain stem dysfunction are found and coma and death supervene if the pressure is not relieved by neurosurgery (craniotomy). **Benign intracranial hypertension** is due to generalised swelling of the brain in the absence of a focal space-occupying lesion. It often occurs in obese young women and the syndrome of raised intracranial pressure mimics a brain tumour, hence the old designation 'pseudo tumour cerebri'.

Foraminal syndromes

The exit foramina of the skull represent sites of potential extrinsic compression of structures running through them, by disorders such as bony deformity and tumours of bone, meninges or blood vessels. The particular cranial nerves damaged at the exit site lead to 'foraminal syndromes', e.g. of the **superior orbital fissure** (see p. 76) or **jugular foramen** (see p. 84). The spinal cord, lower brain stem and the tonsils of the cerebellum are compromised in the **foramen magnum syndrome**.

Skull

- The brain lies on the floor of the cranial cavity, which consists of three fossae.
- The bones of the skull and the meninges provide protection for the brain.
- The anterior cranial fossa contains the frontal lobes of the cerebral hemispheres.
- It forms the roof of the orbit and is closely associated with the frontal air sinus.
- The cribriform plate admits the olfactory nerves to the cranial cavity and accommodates the olfactory bulb.
- The middle cranial fossa contains the temporal lobe. In the midline, the hypophyseal fossa holds the pituitary gland.
- A number of foramina provide entry and exit for important blood vessels and cranial nerves (indicated in parentheses):
  - optic canal (optic nerve, ophthalmic artery)
  - superior orbital fissure (oculomotor, trochlear, abducens and ophthalmic division of trigeminal nerves)
  - foramen rotundum (maxillary division of trigeminal nerve)
  - foramen ovale (mandibular division of trigeminal nerve)
  - foramen lacerum (internal carotid artery)
  - foramen spinosum (middle meningeal artery).
- The posterior cranial fossa accommodates the brain stem and cerebellum.
- A number of important structures pass through the foramina of the posterior fossa:
  - foramen magnum (medulla oblongata, vertebral arteries, spinal root of the accessory nerve)
  - hypoglossal canal (hypoglossal nerve)
  - jugular foramen (internal jugular vein, glossopharyngeal, vagus and accessory nerves)
  - internal auditory meatus (facial and vestibulocochlear nerves).

- The **foramen rotundum** opens into the pterygopalatine fossa and carries the maxillary division of the trigeminal nerve.
- The **foramen ovale** carries the large mandibular division of the trigeminal nerve.
- The **foramen lacerum** lies directly beneath the posterior clinoid process. Through this foramen the internal carotid artery enters the cranial cavity.
- The **foramen spinosum** admits the middle meningeal artery.

Posterior cranial fossa

The posterior cranial fossa is formed by the occipital and petrous temporal bones. Anteriorly, in the midline, it forms a steep, smooth slope (the **clivus**) which is continuous with the body of the sphenoid bone, posterior to the hypophyseal fossa. The brain stem rests upon the clivus, the medulla passing through the **foramen magnum** to become continuous with the spinal cord. The foramen magnum also admits the vertebral arteries and the spinal root of the accessory (XI) nerve. In the lateral wall of the foramen magnum lies the **hypoglossal canal** through which the hypoglossal (XII) nerve leaves the cranial cavity. Between the occipital and petrous temporal bones lies the large **jugular foramen** through which pass the internal jugular vein, the glossopharyngeal (IX), vagus (X) and accessory (XI) nerves. In the vertical wall of the petrous temporal bone is located the **internal auditory (acoustic) meatus** which transmits the vestibulocochlear (VIII) and facial (VII) nerves. The cerebellum rests on the floor of the posterior cranial fossa.

CRANIAL MENINGES

DURA MATER

The cranial dura is a tough, fibrous membrane which ensheathes the brain like a loose-fitting bag. In some regions, such as the floor of the cranial cavity and the midline of the cranial roof, the dura is tightly adherent to the interior surface of the skull whilst elsewhere, such as the fronto-parietal area, the two are separated by a narrow extradural space. Two large reflections of dura extend into the cranial cavity and occupy the fissures between major components of the brain (Figs 4.2 and 4.3). In the midline, a vertical sheet of dura, the **falx cerebri**, extends from the cranial roof into the great longitudinal fissure between the cerebral hemispheres. The falx thus has an attached border which adheres to the inner surface of the skull and a free border which lies above the corpus callosum. A horizontal shelf of dura, the **tentorium cerebelli**, extends inwards from the occipito-temporal region of the skull

Optic chiasma ———— Midbrain ———— Tentorium cerebelli ———— Falx cerebri

Fig. 4.2 **Cranial cavity showing the arrangement of the dura mater**.

Tentorium cerebelli   Falx cerebri   Corpus callosum

Occipital lobe   Cerebellum   Medulla   Pons   Pituitary gland

Fig. 4.3 **Median sagittal section of the head, showing the disposition of the brain and meninges**.

to lie between the posterior part of the cerebral hemispheres and the cerebellum in the transverse cerebral fissure. It has a free border which encircles the midbrain, as the brain stem communicates between the posterior and middle cranial fossae. In the midline the tentorium becomes continuous superiorly with the falx cerebri.

ARACHNOID MATER AND PIA MATER

The arachnoid mater is a soft, translucent membrane which, like the dura mater, loosely envelopes the brain (see Fig. 1.6). It is separated from the dura by a narrow subdural space, through which pass veins en route to the venous sinuses (see below and p. 159).

Head trauma

Head trauma, especially due to road traffic accidents, is the commonest cause of death and disability in youth. The injury may be blunt ('closed') or due to a penetrating missile. The skull may be fractured and depressed tearing brain coverings and the brain itself. Displacement and torsion of the brain lead to contusion, tearing of white matter and bleeding into the brain (**intracerebral haematoma**), causing unconsciousness (concussion), neurological and psychological deficits and post-traumatic epilepsy.

Tearing of the middle meningeal artery causes bleeding into the extradural space (**extradural haematoma**).

As the blood clot expands the brain is compressed so that coma supervenes a delayed period of hours after the blow. Without neurosurgical evacuation the rising intracranial pressure causes brain displacement and death.

Tearing of the veins stretching across the subdural space causes gradual seepage of blood, collecting to form a chronic **subdural haematoma** with eventual coma. The delay between the blow and the development of symptoms may be of weeks or months. The elderly are particularly vulnerable and the head injury may be slight and forgotten. Again, surgical removal of the clot is life-saving.

The pia mater is a microscopically thin, delicate and highly vascular membrane which is closely adherent to the surface of the brain, following all its concavities and convexities. Between the pia and arachnoid mater lies the **subarachnoid space**. This contains a filamentous network of connective tissue strands (trabeculae) and is traversed by numerous arteries and veins. It also contains cerebrospinal fluid which is produced by the choroid plexus within the cerebral ventricles (p. 149). Since the arachnoid mater fits loosely round the brain whilst the pia closely follows its surface contours, the subarachnoid space is of greatly varying depth in different regions. Where significant depressions or fissures in the brain are spanned by the arachnoid mater, **subarachnoid cisterns** are formed. Two of these are particularly large:

- The **cisterna magna** lies between the cerebellum and the dorsal surface of the medulla (Fig. 4.4). Into this cistern flows cerebrospinal fluid from the fourth ventricle.
- The **interpeduncular cistern** is located at the base of the brain, where the arachnoid spans the space between the two temporal lobes. This cistern contains the optic chiasma.

Meningitis

Inflammation of the meninges may be due to infection with virus (e.g. lymphocytic choriomeningitis) or bacteria (meningococcal and tuberculous meningitis), other organisms or chemical reaction to injected contrast medium during neuroradiological procedures. Headache, photophobia and vomiting are complained of. The patient is febrile and has neck stiffness on attempts to move the head. Viral and chemical meningitis are normally mild and self-limiting. Bacterial or fungal meningitis, however, leads to damage to cranial nerves and the brain itself and, if untreated, proceeds to raised intracranial pressure, brain displacement and death.

Cerebellar hemisphere

Arachnoid mater covering cisterna magna

Medulla

Fig. 4.4 **Cisterna magna**.

DURAL VENOUS SINUSES

The dura mater is considered to consist of two layers. These are normally closely adherent to one another but, in certain locations, become separated to enclose blood-filled spaces, the dural venous sinuses. Major venous sinuses lie in the attached borders of the falx cerebri and tentorium cerebelli and also on the floor of the cranial cavity. Venous blood from the brain flows into these sinuses. Through a series of interconnecting channels, these in turn drain into the internal jugular vein, via which blood is returned to the general extra-cranial circulation. The dural venous sinuses are described further in Chapter 16 which deals with the blood supply of the central nervous system.

Cranial meninges

- The dura mater is the outermost membrane. Two dural sheets or reflections extend into the cranial cavity:
  - the falx cerebri, lying between the two cerebral hemispheres
  - the tentorium cerebelli, lying between the cerebellum and the occipital lobes of the cerebrum and encircling the midbrain.
- The dura contains a number of venous sinuses which are important in the venous drainage of the brain.
- Important sinuses lie within the falx cerebri, tentorium cerebelli and on the floor of the cranial cavity.
- The middle meningeal layer is the arachnoid mater. Both the dura and arachnoid surround the brain loosely.
- The innermost meningeal layer is the pia mater, which adheres to the surface of the brain. This creates a subarachnoid space of variable depth.
- The subarachnoid space contains cerebrospinal fluid, which is secreted by the choroid plexus within the cerebral ventricles.

Spinal cord

The spinal cord and its associated spinal nerves are of immense functional importance. These structures act to:

• receive afferent fibres from sensory receptors of the trunk and limbs
• control movements of the trunk and limbs
• provide autonomic innervation for most of the viscera.

The internal organisation of the cord permits many functions to operate in an automatic or reflex fashion.

In addition, extensive connections with the brain, through ascending and descending nerve fibre tracts, both convey afferent information to higher centres and mediate their controlling influence over spinal mechanisms.

EXTERNAL FEATURES OF THE SPINAL CORD

TOPOGRAPHICAL ANATOMY

The spinal cord occupies the vertebral (or spinal) canal within the vertebral column, which provides support and protection (Figs 5.1 and 5.2). It is continuous rostrally with the medulla oblongata of the brain stem.

Fig. 5.1 **Transverse section through the thoracic region**.
The diagram shows the relationship between the spinal cord, spinal nerves and vertebral column.

Fig. 5.2 **Magnetic resonance image of the vertebral column and spinal cord in the living subject.**
(Courtesy of Dr. A. Jackson, Department of Diagnostic Radiology, University of Manchester.)

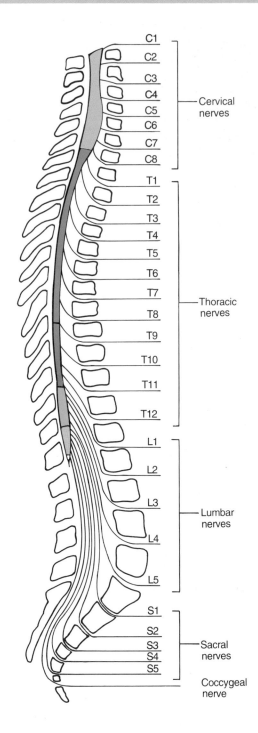

Fig. 5.3 **Schematic representation of the relationships between the spinal cord, spinal nerves and vertebral column.**

The cord is approximately cylindrical in shape but its diameter varies considerably at different levels. It bears two enlargements, cervical and lumbar (Fig. 5.3). The **cervical enlargement** consists of cord segments C3–T1 and provides innervation for the upper limb via the **brachial plexus**. The **lumbar enlargement** (Figs 5.3 and 5.4) is made up of segments L1–S3 and is associated with innervation of the lower limb via the **lumbar plexus** (L1–L4) and the **sacral plexus** (L4–S2). Caudal to the lumbar enlargement, the cord tapers abruptly to form a conical termination, the **conus medullaris**. From the tip of the conus a strand of connective tissue, the **filum terminale** (Fig. 5.4), extends caudally and is attached to the dorsal surface of the first coccygeal vertebra.

Until the third month of fetal life the spinal cord occupies the entire length of the vertebral canal. Thereafter, the rate of elongation of the vertebral column exceeds that of the spinal cord, so that at birth the cord terminates at the level of the third lumbar vertebra (L3) and in adult life at the level of the intervertebral disc between L1 and L2 (Figs 5.3 and 5.4).

The approximate level of spinal cord segments may be identified in the living subject by reference to the posterior spinous processes of the vertebrae. As a rule of thumb, cervical cord segments lie approximately one spine higher than their corresponding vertebrae (e.g. C7 cord segment lies adjacent to C6 vertebra), thoracic segments lie approximately two spines higher and lumbar segments three to four spines higher than their corresponding vertebrae (Fig. 5.3).

Fig. 5.4 **Dorsal aspect of the spinal cord caudal to T9–10**. The dura\arachnoid mater have been cut longitudinally and reflected to reveal the spinal cord and nerve roots within the subarachnoid space.

Labels for Fig. 5.4:
- Denticulate ligament
- Dorsal roots of spinal nerves
- Lumbar enlargement
- Dura mater
- Conus medullaris
- Termination of the spinal cord at L1
- Cauda equina
- Epidural space
- Filum terminale
- Subarachnoid space
- Termination of the subarachnoid space at S2

Labels for Fig. 5.5:
- Pia mater
- Dorsal roots of spinal nerve
- Dorsal root ganglion
- Ventral roots of spinal nerve
- Ventral ramus of spinal nerve
- Denticulate ligament
- Subarachnoid space
- Arachnoid mater
- Dorsal ramus of spinal nerve
- Dura mater

Topographical anatomy

- The spinal cord provides sensory, motor and autonomic innervation for the trunk and limbs.
- The cord possesses two enlargements: cervical (C3–T1) associated with innervation of the upper limbs; lumbar (L1–S3) innervating the lower limbs.
- The cord terminates at vertebral level L1–L2 in the adult.

SPINAL NERVES

The spinal cord bears 31 bilaterally paired spinal nerves (8 cervical, 12 thoracic, 5 lumbar, 5 sacral and 1 coccygeal). These originate as two linear series of nerve fascicles attached to the dorsolateral and ventrolateral aspects of the cord (Fig. 5.5). The groups of 6–8 adjacent fascicles which are attached to each cord segment coalesce to form **dorsal** and **ventral nerve roots**. The dorsal and ventral roots of each cord segment then pass to their corresponding **intervertebral foramen**, in or near which they join to form the spinal nerve proper. Whilst the spinal nerves are mixed nerves, containing both afferent and efferent neurones, the dorsal and ventral roots are functionally distinct. The dorsal roots contain **primary afferent neurones** running from peripheral sensory receptors to the spinal

Fig. 5.5 **Relationships between the spinal cord, spinal nerve roots and the meninges**. (Modified with permission from Carpenter MB, Sutin J 1983 *Human Neuroanatomy*, 8th edn. Williams and Wilkins, Baltimore.)

cord and brain stem. The nerve cell bodies of these neurones are located in **dorsal root ganglia** (Fig. 5.5) which appear as small enlargements on the dorsal roots, near their convergence with the ventral roots at the entrance to the intervertebral foramina. The ventral roots of the spinal nerves carry **efferent neurones** whose cell bodies are located in the spinal grey matter. These comprise motor neurones, which innervate skeletal muscle, and preganglionic neurones of the autonomic nervous system.

C1–C7 spinal nerves exit from the vertebral canal above the first seven cervical vertebrae; C8 spinal nerve exits below the seventh cervical vertebra and the remainder leave below their corresponding vertebrae (Fig. 5.3). Because of the different lengths of the spinal cord and the vertebral canal, only in the cervical region do the spinal cord segments lie adjacent to their corresponding vertebral bodies. Below this level successive spinal nerve roots follow an increasingly oblique downwards course to reach their respective intervertebral foramina. This is most marked for the lumbar and sacral roots which descend below the termination of the cord in a leash-like arrangement, the **cauda equina** (Figs 5.3 and 5.4).

Immediately after leaving the intervertebral foramina, spinal nerves divide to produce a thin **dorsal (posterior) ramus** and a much larger **ventral (anterior) ramus** (Figs 5.1 and 5.5). The dorsal ramus supplies the muscles and skin of the back region. The ventral ramus supplies the muscles and skin of the front of the body and the limbs.

The peripheral distribution of spinal nerves, including their pattern of cutaneous innervation (dermatomes) and innervation of muscle groups (myotomes) is described in Chapter 3.

SPINAL MENINGES

The spinal cord, like the brain, is invested by three concentric meningeal coverings: the pia mater, arachnoid mater and dura mater (Figs 5.4 and 5.5).

The innermost covering, the pia mater, is a delicate, vascular membrane which is closely applied to the surface of the cord and nerve roots. Along a line midway between the dorsal and ventral roots of the spinal nerves is attached a flat, membranous continuation of the pia, called the **denticulate ligament**. The ligament has a free lateral border for much of its length

---

Spinal nerve injury

The spinal nerve roots are vulnerable to compression by degenerative changes in the joints of the spinal column (**spondylosis**) and by **prolapse of intervertebral discs**. Prolapsed intervertebral discs in the cervical spine cause pain in the neck radiating to the arm and hand, accompanied by tingling sensations (paraesthesiae), weakness and wasting of the muscles corresponding to the radicular distribution, numbness of the skin corresponding to the dermatomal distribution, together with loss of the tendon reflexes subserved by the particular root (Fig. 5.6; see also Fig. 1.26). Similarly, lumbar prolapsed intervertebral discs lead to back pain and radiation of pain into the legs, known as **sciatica**. A large lumbosacral prolapsed disc may cause paralysis of the bladder and incontinence, demanding urgent neurosurgery.

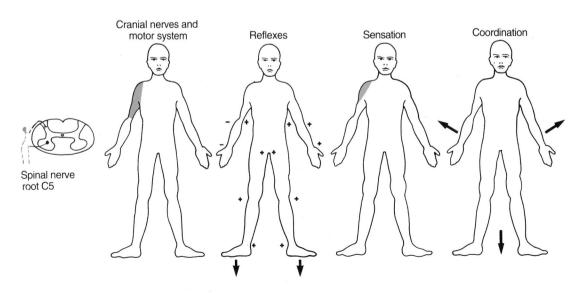

Fig. 5.6 **Spinal nerve root lesion**. *(Key on page 17)*

but, intermittently, lateral projections tether the spinal cord to the arachnoid, and through it to the dura.

The arachnoid mater lies between the pia and dura. It is a translucent membrane which invests the cord like a loose-fitting bag. Between the pia and arachnoid lies the subarachnoid space. This contains cerebrospinal fluid which is produced in the cerebral ventricular system (see p. 149).

The outer covering of the cord, the dura mater, is a tough, fibrous membrane. It envelopes the cord loosely as does the arachnoid, with which it is in contact, though separated by a theoretical plane, the **subdural space**. The dura is separated from the bony wall of the vertebral canal by the **epidural space**.

Although the spinal cord terminates at vertebral level L1–2, the arachnoid and dural sheaths and, thus, the subarachnoid space, continue caudally to S2. As the spinal nerve roots pass towards their intervertebral foramina they evaginate the arachnoid and dura, forming meningeal root sleeves which extend as far as the fusion of dorsal and ventral roots. Thereafter, the arachnoid and dura become continuous with the epineurium ensheathing the spinal nerve.

Lumbar puncture and epidural anaesthesia

The lowest part of the spinal canal does not contain the spinal cord, so that hollow needles can be safely inserted into the subarachnoid space in order to remove cerebrospinal fluid for diagnostic purposes (**lumbar puncture**) or to inject radio-opaque substances for the radiological delineation of the spinal canal and its contents (**myelography**). Similarly, anaesthetics may be introduced into the epidural space in surgical procedures (**epidural block**).

Spinal nerves and meninges

- 31 pairs of spinal nerves attach to the spinal cord as dorsal and ventral roots. Dorsal roots carry afferent fibres; ventral roots carry efferent fibres.
- Spinal nerves exit the vertebral canal via intervertebral foramina.
- Below the termination of the cord, spinal nerve roots descend as the cauda equina.
- The cord and nerve roots are susceptible to traumatic injury, e.g. prolapsed intervertebral disc, cervical spondylosis, spinal dislocation.
- The cord is invested by three meninges (pia, arachnoid and dura mater).
- The subarachnoid space contains cerebrospinal fluid.
- CSF may be removed by lumbar puncture at L2–L3 or L3–L4.
- Epidural anaesthesia of lumbar and sacral spinal nerves is possible at the same level.

INTERNAL STRUCTURE OF THE SPINAL CORD

The spinal cord is incompletely divided into two symmetrical halves by a **dorsal median sulcus** and a **ventral median fissure** (Fig. 5.7). In the centre of the cord is the small **central canal** which is continuous rostrally with the cerebral ventricular system. Surrounding the central canal is the spinal **grey matter** consisting of nerve cell bodies, their dendrites and synaptic contacts. The outer part of the cord consists of **white matter** which contains ascending and descending nerve fibres. Some serve to join neighbouring

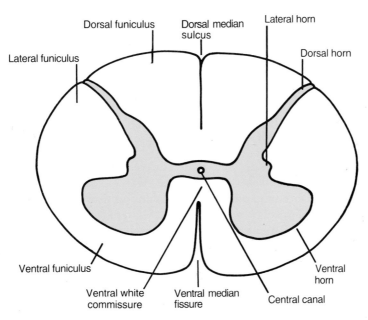

Fig. 5.7 **Schematic transverse section through the spinal cord showing the general disposition of grey and white matter.**

and distant cord segments for the integration of their functions whilst others run between the cord and the brain. Many of the fibres which share a common origin, course and termination are grouped together in fascicles, forming the long **tracts** of the spinal cord.

Different cord levels vary in the relative amounts and configuration of grey and white matter (Fig. 5.8). Higher levels contain greater amounts of white matter. This is because ascending tracts gain fibres at each successive level whereas the opposite is true of descending tracts.

GREY MATTER OF THE SPINAL CORD

The grey matter is approximately H-shaped, or butterfly-shaped, with four protrusions, the dorsal (posterior) and ventral (anterior) horns, extending dorso- and ventrolaterally towards the attachment zones of the dorsal and ventral root fascicles, respectively. The size and shape of the dorsal and ventral horns varies according to the level (Fig. 5.8). Many afferent nerve fibres entering in the dorsal roots terminate in the dorsal horn, whilst the ventral horn contains the cell bodies of motor neurones which exit through the ventral nerve roots and innervate skeletal muscle. Both dorsal and ventral horns are, therefore, particularly well developed at cervical and lumbar levels in association with innervation of the upper and lower limbs. Thoracic and upper lumbar segments additionally possess a small **lateral** or **intermediolateral horn**, located between the dorsal and ventral horns, which contains the cell bodies of **preganglionic sympathetic neurones** (Figs 5.7 and 5.8).

The grey matter of the spinal cord may be divided, on the basis of its cytoarchitecture, into ten zones, **Rexed's laminae**, which are numbered sequentially from dorsal to ventral (Fig. 5.9). Some of these laminae are equated with cell groupings of particular functional types.

Dorsal horn

Afferent fibres entering through the dorsal roots divide into ascending and descending branches. They mostly terminate near their point of entry but may travel for varying distances in either direction, running in the **dorsolateral fasciculus** or **Lissauer's tract** which is located superficial to the tip of the dorsal horn (see Fig. 5.13) and, thus, establishing synaptic contacts over several segments of spinal grey matter. Dorsal root fibres terminate extensively within the grey matter but most densely in the dorsal horn. Cutaneous afferents tend to terminate in superficial (dorsal) laminae whilst proprioceptive and muscle afferents project mostly to deeper laminae.

The tip of the dorsal horn, approximating to Rexed's laminae I–III, is also known as the **substantia gelatinosa**. This region receives collaterals of the smallest diameter myelinated (Group A delta) and unmyelinated (Group C) afferents which are associated with nociception. These neurones are excitatory and use glutamic acid and the peptide substance P as neurotransmitters. In the substantia gelatinosa, complex interactions occur with other types of afferent terminals, interneurones, and with descending pathways from the brain, which control the transmission of pain information to ascending spinothalamic and spinoreticular tract neurones distributed throughout the dorsal horn. For example, input from large diameter afferents carrying tactile information is thought to inhibit transmission of nociceptive impulses to ascending tract neurones, which may explain why rubbing a sore spot can relieve pain.

The substantia gelatinosa contains high levels of the endogenous opioid peptide, enkephalin, which is thought to act as a transmitter of some dorsal horn interneurones. These establish presynaptic contacts with the terminals of primary afferent neurones, which possess opiate receptors. Occupation of these receptors decreases the release of substance P. The analgesic properties of opiates such as morphine are partly due to an action at this site.

Deeper in the dorsal horn, lamina VII contains a number of important cell groups. At cord levels C8–L3, lie the cells of **Clarke's column** (thoracic nucleus, nucleus dorsalis) which are the origin of ascending fibres of the dorsal spinocerebellar tract. The cells of Clarke's column receive afferent input from muscle spindles, Golgi tendon organs, tactile and pressure receptors. At thoracic and upper lumbar levels, the lateral part of lamina VII also contains preganglionic sympathetic neurones which constitute the lateral horn, whilst at sacral levels (S2–S4) it contains preganglionic parasympathetic neurones.

Ventral horn

In the ventral horn, lamina IX corresponds to groups of motor neurones which innervate skeletal muscle. These are of two types:

- **alpha motor neurones** innervate extrafusal muscle fibres
- **gamma motor neurones** innervate intrafusal muscle fibres (within muscle spindles).

The ventral horn is particularly well developed in the cervical and lumbar enlargements due to the presence of motor neurones innervating the upper and lower limbs. Generally speaking, neurones innervating axial musculature (neck and trunk) tend to be located medially whilst those innervating limb muscles are positioned more laterally. In the ventral horn of cord segments C3–C5 is located the **phrenic nucleus**, a group of motor neurones which innervate the diaphragm via the phrenic nerve and are, thus, essential for breathing. Cells in the ventral horn receive direct input from

Fig. 5.9 **Lamination of spinal grey matter (Rexed's laminae).**

Fig. 5.8 **Transverse sections through the spinal cord at cervical, thoracic, lumbar and sacral levels.**
The histological method employed (Weigert-Pal) stains white matter (myelinated nerve fibres), leaving grey matter (nerve cell bodies) relatively unstained.

certain dorsal root afferents (e.g. from muscle spindles for mediation of the stretch reflex). Importantly, they also receive input from pathways descending from higher centres concerned with motor control.

SPINAL REFLEXES

A reflex is an involuntary, stereotyped pattern of response brought about by a sensory stimulus. Although the qualitative nature of an established reflex response is constant it may vary considerably in a quantitative

Grey matter of the spinal cord

- Internally, the spinal cord consists of a central core of grey matter (cell bodies) and an outer mantle of white matter (nerve fibres).
- Within the grey matter, the dorsal horn is the main site of termination of primary afferent fibres. It includes the substantia gelatinosa which is important in transmission of nociceptive impulses to the brain.
- The lateral horn contains preganglionic sympathetic neurones.
- The ventral horn contains alpha and gamma motor neurones, also known as lower motor neurones.

sense (e.g. in delay, duration and extent) due to inter-segmental and supraspinal influences.

Anatomically, the pathways mediating reflex actions consist of afferent neurones conveying impulses from sensory receptors to the CNS (spinal cord or brain stem) and efferent neurones running from the CNS to the effector organ (muscle or gland). In all but the simplest reflexes, interneurones within the CNS are interposed between the afferent and efferent components. The internal organisation of the spinal cord (and brain stem) thus subserves a number of more or less complex reflex functions, some of which are both relatively well understood and clinically important.

Stretch reflex

If a muscle is stretched it responds by contracting and this is known as the **stretch** or **myotatic reflex**. Anatomically this is the simplest of reflexes and is mediated by a **monosynaptic reflex arc** (Fig. 5.10). It consists of afferent neurones which convey impulses from muscle stretch receptors to the CNS and motor neurones which convey impulses back to the stretched muscle.

Stretch receptors within muscles consist of sensory nerve endings which attach to the central, non-contractile region of specialised muscle cells, called **intrafusal muscle fibres**. Intrafusal muscle fibres are oriented parallel to the long axis of the main muscle and occur in groups called **muscle spindles**. Stretch applied to the muscle in which they lie stimulates the sensory endings. Their afferent fibres carry impulses to the CNS, where they make monosynaptic excitatory contact with alpha motor neurones which innervate the bulk of the muscle (**extrafusal muscle fibres**) and make it contract.

There are two types of intrafusal muscle fibre: **nuclear bag** and **nuclear chain** fibres. These bear two types of sensory ending:

- the **primary** or **annulospiral ending**, associated with Group Ia afferent fibres,
- the **secondary** or **flower-spray ending**, associated with Group II afferents.

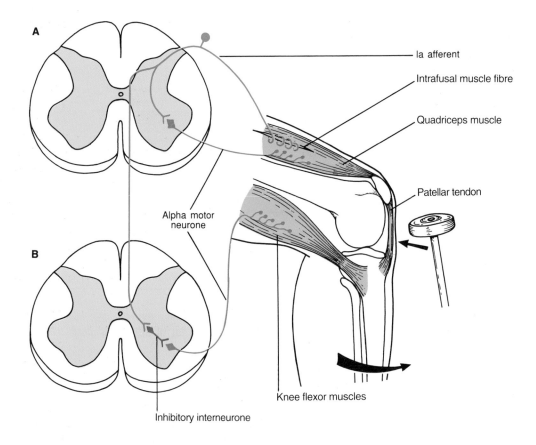

Fig. 5.10 The stretch reflex and reciprocal innervation.
(**A**) The quadriceps stretch reflex is illustrated, whereby striking the patellar tendon elicits extension of the knee. (**B**) Reciprocal innervation: whilst stretching of the quadriceps muscle causes its reflex contraction, the motor neurones of antagonistic muscles (knee flexors) are inhibited by interneuronal connections within the spinal cord.

When a muscle is stretched these endings are stimulated. Primary endings have both velocity and length sensitivity whilst secondary endings have essentially only length sensitivity. Group Ia afferents from a particular muscle make excitatory monosynaptic contact with alpha motor neurones innervating the same muscle, and thus mediate the myotatic reflex.

Stretch reflexes are important in the control of skeletal muscle tone, which refers to the degree of resistance to passive movement, and is determined by the proportion of motor units which are active at any one time. When the upper motor neurones (p. 54) are damaged muscle tone is increased during initial muscle stretch (spasticity). Since stretch reflexes operate to maintain muscles at a constant length in opposition to imposed stretch they are important in the control of posture. By their action activity is maintained in neck, trunk and lower limb extensor muscles (anti-gravity muscles) which support an upright body posture against the force of gravity and are stretched when these body parts become flexed.

In addition to alpha motor neurones which innervate extrafusal muscle fibres, the ventral horn of the spinal cord (and motor cranial nerve nuclei) contain **gamma motor neurones** which innervate the polar, contractile elements of intrafusal muscle fibres (Fig. 5.11). When gamma motor neurones are activated the resultant contraction of the intrafusal muscle fibre applies tension to the sensory endings. This lowers the threshold of the stretch receptors to externally applied stretch and, thus, increases the sensitivity of the stretch reflex (the **gamma reflex loop**, Fig. 5.11).

Like alpha motor neurones, gamma motor neurones are under the influence of descending pathways from the brain. Abnormalities in the activity of these pathways, therefore, which occur in many pathological conditions, induce changes in the sensitivity of stretch reflexes. This is evidenced by abnormalities in muscle tone.

Fig. 5.11 **Gamma reflex loop**.

When a stretch reflex is elicited (e.g. the quadriceps reflex, by tapping the patellar tendon), primary afferent fibres from the muscle spindle not only excite the alpha motor neurones of the stretched muscle, but also interneurones which inhibit the alpha motor neurones of antagonistic muscles (e.g. the knee flexors, Fig. 5.10). This illustrates the general principle of **reciprocal innervation** of agonist and antagonist muscle groups.

Flexor reflex

Noxious cutaneous stimulation of the limbs causes withdrawal from the offending stimulus. This is mediated by a **polysynaptic reflex** in which one or more interneurones are interposed between afferent and efferent neurones. Primary afferent fibres activate interneurones within the spinal grey matter, which in turn excite alpha motor neurones innervating the limb flexor muscles (Fig. 5.12). Flexion of a limb about several joints requires the coordinated action of more than one spinal segment and this is achieved by collateralisation of primary afferents and interneurones.

All forms of cutaneous stimulation have the potential to elicit the flexor reflex, but this is normally prevented by descending pathways from the brain unless the stimulus is painful. In certain pathological conditions the descending inhibitory influence is lost and even innocuous cutaneous stimulation can cause limb withdrawal. The extensor plantar (Babinski) response is a partial flexion withdrawal of the great toe on stimulation of the sole of the foot.

Activation of the flexor reflex in a weight-bearing limb (e.g. by standing on a pin), simultaneously causes reflex extension of the contralateral limb to take the weight of the body. This is called the **crossed extensor reflex** (Fig. 5.12). It is mediated by axon collaterals of primary afferents from the stimulated area, which cross the midline of the cord and excite the alpha motor neurones of contralateral limb extensor muscles.

Tendon reflexes

Deep tendon reflexes, or tendon jerks, are monosynaptic stretch reflexes, elicited during clinical examination by percussion of the tendon of the muscle, by a tendon hammer. Each tendon reflex is subserved by certain spinal cord segments:

Reflex	Cord segments
Biceps reflex (biceps jerk)	C5/C6
Brachioradialis reflex (supinator jerk)	C5/C6
Triceps reflex (triceps jerk)	C6/C7
Quadriceps reflex (knee jerk)	L3/L4
Achilles tendon reflex (ankle jerk)	S1/S2

Lumbar cord

Interneurone

Cutaneous afferent
neurone

Alpha motor neurones

Quadriceps muscle

Knee flexor
muscles

Fig. 5.12 **Flexor reflex and crossed extensor reflex**.

Spinal reflexes

- The internal organisation of the cord subserves a number of important reflex functions.
- The monosynaptic stretch reflex mediates muscle contraction in response to stretch of muscle spindles.
- The sensitivity of the stretch reflex is regulated by gamma motor neurones which provide motor innervation to the spindle fibres.
- The stretch reflex is responsible for maintenance of muscle tone and is clinically tested as the deep tendon reflexes.

WHITE MATTER OF THE SPINAL CORD

The grey matter of the spinal cord is completely surrounded by white matter, which consists of ascending and descending nerve fibres. The white matter is sometimes considered to be divided into dorsal, lateral and ventral columns or **funiculi** (Fig. 5.7). Nerve fibres sharing common origins, terminations and functions are organised into **tracts** or **fasciculi** (latin: small bundles). Some fibres interconnect adjacent or distant cord segments and permit intersegmental coordination, whilst other fibres are longer and serve to join the spinal cord with the brain. The **intersegmental** or **propriospinal** fibres occupy a narrow band immediately peripheral to the grey matter. This is known as the **fasciculus proprius** (Fig. 5.13). Nerve fibres running between the spinal cord and the brain constitute the **ascending** and **descending tracts** of the spinal cord (Figs 5.13–5.19).

Ascending spinal tracts

Ascending tracts carry impulses from pain, thermal, tactile, muscle and joint receptors to the brain. Some of this information eventually reaches a conscious level (the cerebral cortex) while some is destined for subconscious centres (e.g. the cerebellum).

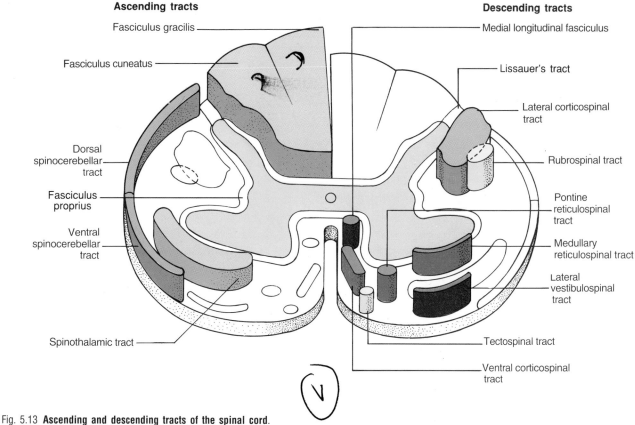

Ascending tracts

Fasciculus gracilis

Fasciculus cuneatus

Dorsal spinocerebellar tract

Fasciculus proprius

Ventral spinocerebellar tract

Spinothalamic tract

Descending tracts

Medial longitudinal fasciculus

Lissauer's tract

Lateral corticospinal tract

Rubrospinal tract

Pontine reticulospinal tract

Medullary reticulospinal tract

Lateral vestibulospinal tract

Tectospinal tract

Ventral corticospinal tract

Fig. 5.13 **Ascending and descending tracts of the spinal cord.**
All ascending and descending tracts are present bilaterally. In this figure, ascending tracts are emphasised on the left side and descending tracts are emphasised on the right side. In addition, the locations of Lissauer's tract and the fasciculus proprius (which contain both ascending and descending fibres) are shown.

Pathways which carry information to a conscious level share certain common characteristics:

- There is a sequence of three neurones between the peripheral receptor and the cerebral cortex.
- The first neurone (first-order neurone or primary afferent neurone) enters the cord through the dorsal root of a spinal nerve and its cell body lies in the dorsal root ganglion. The central process may collateralise extensively and make synaptic connections which mediate spinal reflexes and intersegment coordination. The main fibre remains on the ipsilateral side of the cord and terminates in synaptic contact with the second neurone either in the spinal grey matter or in the medulla oblongata of the brain stem.
- The second neurone (second-order neurone) has its cell body in the cord or medulla oblongata. Its axon crosses over (decussates) to the opposite side of the CNS and ascends to the thalamus, where it terminates upon the third neurone.
- The third-order neurone has its cell body in the thalamus. Its axon passes to the somatosensory cortex of the parietal lobe of the cerebral hemisphere.

Two main tract systems in the spinal cord fit into this pattern: the dorsal (posterior) columns and the spinothalamic tracts.

Dorsal columns

The dorsal columns are located between the dorsal median sulcus and the dorsal horn. Two tracts are recognised:

- the **fasciculus gracilis**, situated medially
- the **fasciculus cuneatus**, situated laterally.

The tracts carry impulses concerned with proprioception (movement and joint position sense) and discriminative touch.

The dorsal columns contain the axons of primary afferent neurones which have entered the cord through the dorsal roots of spinal nerves (Fig. 5.14). The fasciculus gracilis consists of fibres which join the cord at sacral, lumbar and lower thoracic levels whilst fibres of the fasciculus cuneatus enter via the upper thoracic and cervical dorsal roots. Since they contain primary afferent neurones the dorsal columns carry information relating to the ipsilateral side of the body. Fibres ascend without interruption to the medulla oblongata where they terminate upon second-order neurones whose cell bodies are located in the **nucleus gracilis** and **nucleus cuneatus**.

The axons of second-order neurones decussate in the medulla as **internal arcuate fibres** and thereafter ascend through the brain stem as the **medial**

Leg area

Sensory cortex

Arm area

Cerebral hemisphere

Caudate nucleus

Internal capsule

VP thalamus

Putamen

Midbrain
- Medial lemniscus
- Red nucleus
- Substantia nigra
- Crus cerebri

Pons
- Medial leminiscus
- Middle cerebellar peduncle

Medulla
- Nucleus gracilis
- Nucleus cuneatus
- Internal arcuate fibres
- Medial lemniscus
- Pyramid

Cervical cord

Lumbar cord

Fig. 5.14 **The dorsal columns system**.
The central pathways carrying conscious proprioception and discriminative touch are illustrated.

Lesions of the dorsal columns

Tabes dorsalis is a late manifestation of syphilitic infection of the central nervous system. It chiefly affects the lumbosacral dorsal spinal roots and the dorsal columns of the spinal cord. The loss of proprioception leads to a high steppage and unsteady gait (**sensory ataxia**), which is exacerbated when the eyes are closed (**Romberg's sign**).

Subacute combined degeneration of the spinal cord is a systemic disease which results from a deficiency of vitamin B_{12} (cyanocobalamin), which also causes pernicious anaemia. The degeneration of the dorsal columns produces sensory ataxia. The lateral columns of the spinal cord are also involved (combined) causing weakness and spasticity of the limbs. The disorder, although uncommon, is an important one since proper treatment with vitamin B_{12} can lead to complete recovery.

In **multiple sclerosis**, an immune disease, specific damage to the fasciculus cuneatus of the cervical spinal cord leads to loss of proprioception in the hands and fingers, causing profound loss of dexterity and inability to identify the shape and nature of objects by touch alone (**astereognosis**).

Cerebral hemisphere

Leg area

Sensory cortex

Arm area

Internal capsule

VP thalamus

Midbrain

Spinal lemniscus

Pons

Medulla

Cervical cord

Lumbar cord

Fig. 5.15 **The spinothalamic tract system.**
The central pathways for pain, temperature, touch and pressure
are illustrated.

lemniscus. The medial lemniscus terminates in the
ventral posterior (VP) nucleus of the thalamus upon
third-order thalamocortical neurones which project to
the somatosensory cortex.

Spinothalamic tract

The spinothalamic tract lies lateral and ventral to the
ventral horn of the spinal grey matter. It carries information related to pain and thermal sensations and also
non-discriminative touch and pressure. Some author-
ities identify distinct lateral and ventral spinothalamic
tracts conveying pain and temperature or touch and
pressure, respectively, but fibres carrying these
modalities are probably intermingled, at least to some
extent.

The spinothalamic tract contains second-order neurones whose cell bodies of origin lie in the contralateral
dorsal horn and receive input from primary afferent
fibres which terminate in this region (Fig. 5.15). After
leaving the parent cell bodies, spinothalamic axons
decussate to the opposite side of the cord by passing
through the **ventral white commissure,** which lies
ventral to the central canal of the cord, and, thus, enter
the contralateral spinothalamic tract. Axons carrying
pain and temperature decussate within one segment of
their origin, whilst those carrying touch and pressure
may ascend for several segments before decussation.

The spinothalamic tracts can be selectively damaged in **syringomyelia**, in which the central canal becomes enlarged to form a cavity compressing adjacent nerve fibres. The second-order neurones subserving pain and temperature are damaged as they decussate in the ventral white commissure, close to the central canal, causing a selective loss of pain and temperature in the upper limbs. This is termed a **dissociated sensory loss**, since light touch and proprioceptive sensation are retained. The patient injures and burns the hands painlessly and joints of the limbs become disorganised without discomfort (**Charcot joints**).

Selective surgical destruction of the spinothalamic tracts (**cordotomy** or **tractotomy**) is sometimes performed for the neurosurgical relief of intractable pain due to a variety of causes.

Friedreich's ataxia

Friedreich's ataxia is an inherited degenerative disease in which the spinocerebellar tracts are particularly disordered, leading to profound incoordination of the arms (intention tremor) and a wide-based, reeling gait (ataxia). The disorder begins in childhood and the patient is wheelchair-bound by 20 years of age.

In the brain stem the spinothalamic fibres run in proximity to the medial lemniscus and are known as the **spinal lemniscus**. The majority of fibres terminate in the ventral posterior nucleus (VP) of the thalamus, contacting third-order thalamocortical neurones which project to the somatosensory cortex.

The spinothalamic tract is sometimes referred to as the neospinothalamic system. It is highly organised somatotopically so that the origin of sensory stimuli can be accurately localised. It is thought to be the route via which sharp, pricking pain (sometimes called 'fast' pain) is conducted.

The **spinoreticulothalamic system** represents an additional, phylogenetically older, route by which sensory impulses ascend to higher centres. Some second-order neurones arising from the dorsal horn ascend in the ventrolateral region of the cord and then terminate in the brain stem reticular formation, particularly within the medulla. Reticulothalamic fibres then ascend to the intralaminar thalamic nuclei, which in turn activate the cerebral cortex. The spinoreticulothalamic system is thought to be the route via which dull, aching pain (sometimes called 'slow pain') is transmitted to a conscious level. Activation of spinothalamic and spinoreticular fibres, which may ultimately be perceived as unpleasant or painful, can be modulated by descending pathways from the brain.

Ascending pathways which carry impulses to a subconscious level are represented by the spinocerebellar tracts.

Spinocerebellar tracts

Fibres of this ascending system constitute the dorsal and ventral spinocerebellar tracts, which are located near the dorsolateral and ventrolateral surfaces of the cord, respectively. Both tracts carry information de-

rived from muscle spindles, Golgi tendon organs and tactile receptors to the cerebellum for the control of posture and coordination of movement.

The spinocerebellar system consists of a sequence of only two neurones. Both spinocerebellar tracts contain second-order neurones whose cell bodies of origin lie in the base of the dorsal horn and receive input from primary afferent fibres terminating in this region. The tract neurones terminate directly in the cerebellar cortex, predominantly within the vermis. Fibres of the dorsal spinocerebellar tract originate from a prominent group of cells known as **Clarke's column**. The axons ascend ipsilaterally to enter the cerebellum through the **inferior cerebellar peduncle**. Fibres of the ventral spinocerebellar tract decussate, ascend on the contralateral side of the cord and enter the cerebellum via the **superior cerebellar peduncle**. Some axons then recross within the cerebellar white matter.

White matter of the spinal cord – principal ascending tracts

- Ascending tracts carry afferent information to conscious and subconscious levels. Pathways to a conscious level follow a basic plan of three neurones in a chain from peripheral receptor to cerebral cortex.
- Dorsal columns (fasciculus gracilis and cuneatus) carry proprioception and discriminative touch. They convey first-order neurones ipsilaterally to the nuclei gracilis and cuneatus of the medulla. Second-order neurones decussate and pass to the thalamus. Third-order neurones project to the somatosensory cortex. Lesions (e.g. tabes dorsalis, vitamin B_{12} deficiency) lead to ataxia and loss of discriminative touch.
- Spinothalamic tract carries pain, temperature, touch and pressure sensations. The tract contains second-order neurones with cell bodies in the dorsal horn. Axons decussate and pass to the thalamus. Third-order neurones project to the somatosensory cortex. Lesions (e.g. syringomyelia) lead to impairment of pain, temperature, touch and pressure sensitivity on the contralateral side.
- Dorsal and ventral spinocerebellar tracts contain second-order neurones carrying muscle, joint and tactile information involved in motor control. Lesions lead to ataxia (e.g. Friedreich's ataxia).

Leg area

Motor Cortex

**Cerebral
hemisphere**

Arm area

**Periaqueductal
grey**

Midbrain

Pons

**Fascicles of
corticospinal
fibres**

Medulla

Pyramid

**Decussation
of the
pyramids**

Cervical cord

**Lateral
corticospinal
tract**

Ventral
corticospinal
tract

Lumbar cord

Fig. 5.16 **Corticospinal tracts**.

Descending spinal tracts

Descending tracts of the spinal cord (Fig. 5.13) originate from the cerebral cortex and brain stem. They are concerned with the control of movement, muscle tone, spinal reflexes, spinal autonomic functions and the transmission of sensory information to higher centres.

Corticospinal tracts

The corticospinal tracts (Fig. 5.16) are particularly concerned with the control of voluntary, discrete, skilled movements, sometimes referred to as 'fractionated movements', and especially those of the distal parts of the limbs. Corticospinal tract neurones arise from cell bodies in the cerebral cortex. The cells of origin are widely distributed in the motor and sensory cortices, including the **precentral gyrus** or **primary motor cortex**, where the large **Betz cells** give rise to the largest diameter corticospinal axons. Corticospinal axons leave the cerebral hemispheres by passing through the

Hereditary spastic paraparesis

Hereditary spastic paraparesis is an inherited degenerative disorder (autosomal dominant) in which progressive weakness affects the legs leading to marked stiffness of gait. Degeneration of the lateral columns, including the lateral corticospinal tract, chiefly affects the thoracic spinal cord causing a spastic paraparesis with hyperreflexia and extensor plantar responses, but with sparing of sensation and bladder function.

massive subcortical fibre systems of the **corona radiata** and **internal capsule** to enter the **crus cerebri** of the midbrain.

Having passed through the ventral portion of the pons, corticospinal fibres reach the medulla oblongata, where they form two prominent columns on the ventral surface. These are called the **pyramids** and for this reason the term **pyramidal tract** is used as an alternative name for the corticospinal tract. In the caudal medulla the fibres of the pyramids undergo subtotal decussation. About 75–90% of fibres decussate and enter the contralateral **lateral corticospinal tract** which is located in the lateral part of the spinal white matter, deep to the dorsal spinocerebellar tract; 10–25% of pyramidal fibres remain ipsilateral and enter the **ventral corticospinal tract**, located lateral to the ventral median fissure. They also decussate near to their termination, so that the fibres of the pyramidal tract effectively innervate the contralateral side of the spinal cord.

About 55% of corticospinal neurones terminate at cervical levels, 20% at thoracic and 25% at lumbosacral levels. Fibres terminate extensively in the spinal grey matter. Many of those fibres which originate from the motor cortex terminate in the ventral horn, some making monosynaptic contact with motor neurones.

Rubrospinal tract

The rubrospinal tract originates from the **red nucleus** of the midbrain tegmentum (Fig. 5.17). It exerts control over the tone of limb flexor muscles, being excitatory to the motor neurones of these muscles. Axons leaving the cells of the red nucleus course ventromedially and cross in the **ventral tegmental decussation**, after which they descend to the spinal cord where they lie ventrolateral to, and partly intermingled with, the lateral corticospinal tract.

The red nucleus receives afferent fibres from the motor cortex and from the cerebellum. The rubrospinal tract thus represents a non-pyramidal route by which the motor cortex and cerebellum can influence spinal motor activity.

Tectospinal tract

Tectospinal fibres arise from the **superior colliculus** of the midbrain (Fig. 5.18). Axons pass ventromedially around the periaqueductal grey matter and cross in the **dorsal tegmental decussation**. In the spinal cord descending tectospinal fibres lie near the ventral median fissure and terminate predominantly in cervical segments. The superior colliculus receives visual input and the tectospinal tract is thought to mediate reflex movements in response to visual stimuli.

Vestibulospinal tracts

Vestibulospinal fibres arise from the **vestibular nuclei** situated in the pons and medulla, in and near the floor of the fourth ventricle (Fig. 5.19). The vestibular nuclei receive input from the labyrinthine system by way of the vestibular nerve and from the cerebellum.

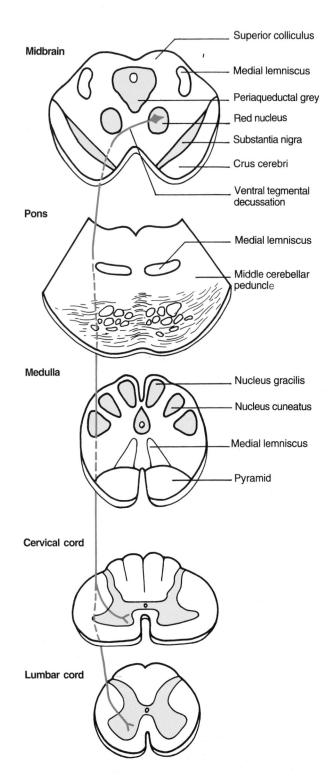

Midbrain

Superior colliculus

Medial lemniscus

Periaqueductal grey

Red nucleus

Substantia nigra

Crus cerebri

Ventral tegmental decussation

Pons

Medial lemniscus

Middle cerebellar peduncle

Medulla

Nucleus gracilis

Nucleus cuneatus

Medial lemniscus

Pyramid

Cervical cord

Lumbar cord

Fig. 5.17 **Rubrospinal tract**.

Fig. 5.18 **Tectospinal tract**.

Fig. 5.19 **Vestibulospinal tracts**.

Axons from cells of the **lateral vestibular nucleus (Deiters' nucleus)** descend ipsilaterally as the **lateral vestibulospinal tract** which is located in the ventral funiculus. Lateral vestibulospinal tract fibres mediate excitatory influences upon extensor motor neurones. They serve to control extensor muscle tone in the anti-gravity maintenance of posture.

The **medial vestibular nucleus** contributes descending fibres to the ipsilateral **medial longitudinal fasciculus** (MLF), also known as the **medial vestibulospinal tract**, which is located adjacent to the ventral median fissure.

Reticulospinal tracts

The reticular formation of the pons and medulla gives rise to reticulospinal fibres. Axons arising from the pontine reticular formation descend ipsilaterally as the **medial** (or **pontine**) **reticulospinal tract**. Axons from the medulla descend bilaterally in the **lateral** (or **medullary**) **reticulospinal tracts**. Both tracts are located in the ventral funiculus.

Reticulospinal fibres influence voluntary movement, reflex activity and muscle tone by controlling the activity of both alpha and gamma motor neurones. They also mediate pressor and depressor effects upon the circulatory system and are involved in the control of breathing.

White matter of the spinal cord – principal descending tracts

- Corticospinal tract controls discrete, skilled movements particularly of the distal extremities. It originates from motor and sensory cortices. Fibres descend through the internal capsule, crus cerebri and ventral pons to reach the medullary pyramid. 75–90% of fibres decussate to form the lateral corticospinal tract, the remainder forming the ventral corticospinal tract.
- Rubrospinal tract controls limb flexor muscles and originates from the red nucleus of the midbrain. Fibres cross in the ventral tegmental decussation.
- Tectospinal tract is involved in reflex responses to visual input. It originates from the contralateral superior colliculus and fibres cross in the dorsal tegmental decussation.
- Vestibulospinal tracts descend from the vestibular nuclei. The lateral vestibulospinal tract originates from the ipsilateral lateral vestibular nucleus and mediates excitation of limb extensor muscles.
- Reticulospinal tracts descend from the pons and medulla. They are involved in the control of reflex activities, muscle tone and vital functions.

Lower and upper motor neurone lesions

The motor neurones of the cord (and brain stem), and their axonal processes, are referred to clinically as **lower motor neurones**. This distinguishes them from the neurones and axons of the descending tracts, which control the activity of spinal and brain stem neurones, and which are themselves collectively referred to as **upper motor neurones**.

The descending tract cells can be damaged at many locations within the CNS and by many different pathologies. Individual tracts are rarely damaged in isolation and, thus, it is often difficult to attribute clinical deficits to involvement of particular pathways. Generally speaking, however, upper motor neurone lesions are associated with a number of motor signs and symptoms which distinguishes them from damage to the lower motor neurone. The distinction between upper and lower motor neurone syndromes is critical in neurological examination and diagnosis.

Lower motor neurone syndrome
- Weakness (paresis) or paralysis (plegia) of individual muscles.
- Wasting of muscles.
- Visible spontaneous contractions of motor units (fasciculation).
- Reduced resistance to passive stretching (hypotonia).
- Diminution or loss of deep tendon reflexes (hyporeflexia or areflexia).

Upper motor neurone syndrome
- Weakness or paralysis of specific movements (extension of the upper limbs and flexion of the lower limbs, termed 'pyramidal weakness').
- No wasting of muscles.
- Increased resistance to passive stretching of muscles (spasticity).
- Hyperactivity of deep tendon reflexes (hyperreflexia).
- Emergence of the extensor plantar response (positive **Babinski reflex**) leading to dorsiflexion of the great toe on stimulation of the sole of the foot.

The lower motor neurones of the spinal cord may be selectively affected by two diseases. **Poliomyelitis** is an acute viral infection of the neurones leading to rapid paralysis and wasting of the limb and respiratory muscles. The disability is often asymmetrical and frequently affects the legs. Recovery occurs but may be incomplete. **Motor neurone disease** is a chronic degenerative disorder which affects both lower motor neurones and the descending tracts to the spinal cord (upper motor neurones). Degeneration of ventral horn cells causes weakness, wasting, hypotonia and fasciculation of the limb muscles (**progressive muscular atrophy**). Degeneration of descending pathways leads to weakness and spasticity of the limb muscles (**amyotrophic lateral sclerosis**).

The clinical signs of upper motor neurone dysfunction are often referred to as 'pyramidal signs' which implies that they are due solely to damage to the pyramidal tract. This is not usually the case. Damage to the pyramidal tract itself probably accounts for the loss of discrete movements and the appearance of the Babinski reflex. Hyperreflexia and spasticity are due to the involvement of other pathways. Descending pathways which influence muscle tone, posture and movement, other than the corticospinal or pyramidal tracts, are sometimes referred to collectively as **extrapyramidal** pathways.

Lesions of the spinal cord

Focal lesions of the spinal cord and the nerve roots produce clinical manifestations in two ways:

- the lesion destroys function at the segmental level
- the lesion interrupts descending motor and ascending sensory tracts.

Damage to different parts of the spinal cord, therefore, is accompanied by distinctive clinical syndromes, which can be diagrammatically represented (Fig. 5.20A-E; see also Fig. 1.26, p. 17).

Upper cervical cord lesion. A high cervical cord lesion causes spastic tetraplegia with hyperreflexia, extensor plantar responses (upper motor neurone lesion), incontinence, sensory loss below the level of the lesion and 'sensory' ataxia (Fig. 5.20A).

Lower cervical cord lesion. A lower cervical cord lesion causes weakness, wasting and fasciculation of muscles, and areflexia of the upper limbs (lower motor neurone lesion). In addition, there is spastic paraparesis, hyperreflexia and extensor plantar responses (upper motor neurone lesion) in the lower limbs, incontinence, sensory loss below the level of the lesion and 'sensory' ataxia (Fig. 5.20B).

Thoracic cord lesion. A thoracic cord lesion causes a spastic paraparesis, hyperreflexia and extensor plantar responses (upper motor neurone lesion), incontinence, sensory loss below the level of the lesion and 'sensory' ataxia (Fig. 5.20C).

Lumbar cord lesion. A lumbar cord lesion causes weakness, wasting and fasciculation of muscles, and areflexia of the lower limbs (lower motor neurone lesion), incontinence, sensory loss below the level of the lesion and 'sensory' ataxia (Fig. 5.20D).

Hemisection of the cord gives rise to the **Brown–Sequard syndrome** (Fig. 5.20E). This is characterised by ipsilateral loss of proprioception and upper motor neurone signs (hemiplegia\monoplegia) plus contralateral loss of pain and temperature sensation.

(continued overleaf)

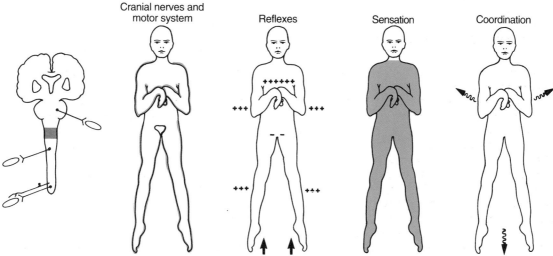

Fig. 5.20A **Upper cervical cord lesion**.

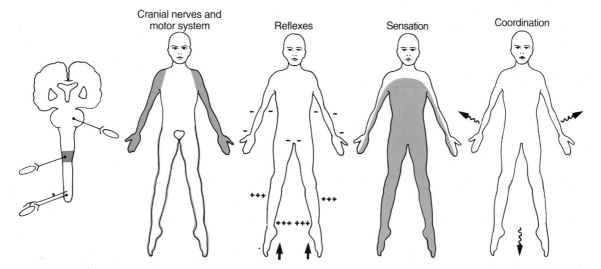

Fig. 5.20B **Lower cervical cord lesion**.

(Key on page 17)

Lesions of spinal cord (*continued*)

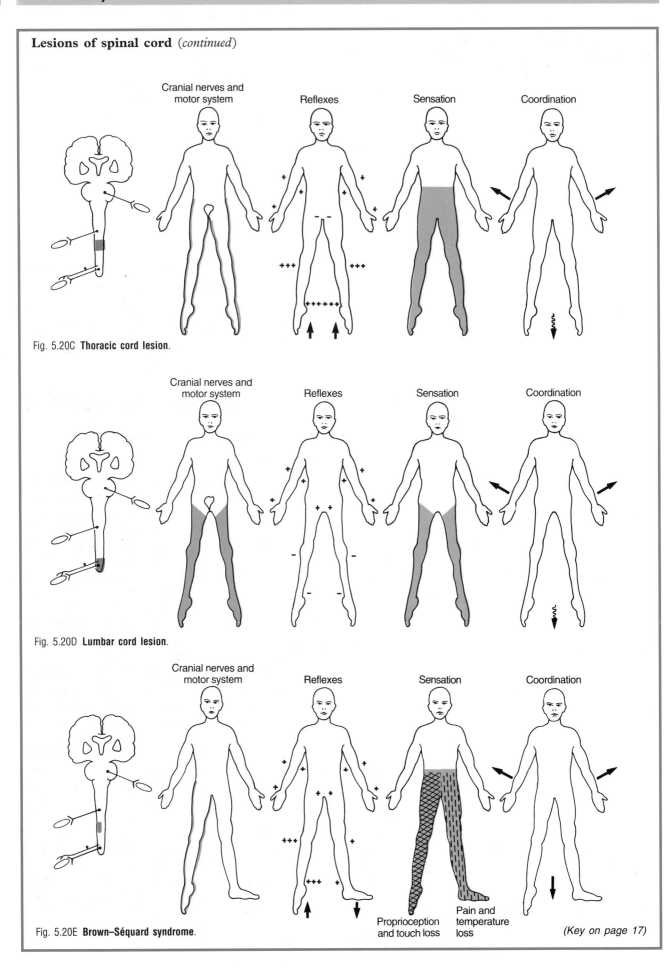

Cranial nerves and motor system   Reflexes   Sensation   Coordination

Fig. 5.20C **Thoracic cord lesion**.

Cranial nerves and motor system   Reflexes   Sensation   Coordination

Fig. 5.20D **Lumbar cord lesion**.

Cranial nerves and motor system   Reflexes   Sensation   Coordination

Fig. 5.20E **Brown–Séquard syndrome**.

Proprioception and touch loss

Pain and temperature loss

(Key on page 17)

Brain stem

The brain stem consists of the medulla oblongata, pons and midbrain. The archaic term 'bulb' is applied to the brain stem in compound anatomical names given to nerve fibres originating from, or terminating in, the brain stem (e.g. 'corticobulbar' refers to axons which arise in the cerebral cortex and terminate in the brain stem). It is also used clinically to denote the medulla in such terms as 'bulbar palsy' and 'pseudobulbar palsy' which describe syndromes associated with medullary dysfunction. The brain stem lies upon the basal portion of the occipital bone (clivus) and is connected to, and largely covered by, the cerebellum. Caudally, the medulla is continuous with the spinal cord at the level of the foramen magnum. Rostrally, the midbrain is continuous with the diencephalon of the forebrain.

The brain stem contains numerous ascending and descending fibre tracts. Some of these pass throughout its whole length, having their origin in the spinal cord or cerebral hemisphere, respectively; others have their origin or termination within brain stem nuclei. Certain nuclei receive fibres from, or send fibres into, cranial nerves, ten pairs of which (III–XII) attach to the surface of the brain stem. These are known as the **cranial nerve nuclei**. In addition, the brain stem contains a complex and heterogeneous matrix of neurones known as the **reticular formation**, within which a number of individually identified nuclei exist. The reticular formation has a number of important functions, including control over the level of consciousness, the perception of pain and regulation of the cardiovascular and respiratory systems. It also has extensive connections with the cranial nerve nuclei, the cerebellum and with brain stem and spinal motor mechanisms through which it influences movement, posture and muscle tone.

EXTERNAL FEATURES OF THE BRAIN STEM

DORSAL SURFACE OF THE BRAIN STEM
(Figs 6.1 and 6.3)

The dorsal surface of the brain stem can be viewed if the overlying cerebellum is removed by cutting the three pairs of **peduncles**, or nerve fibre bundles, by which it is attached on each side. On the dorsal surface of the medulla, the midline is marked by a dorsal median sulcus, continuous with that of the spinal cord. In the caudal part of the medulla, the **dorsal columns** (**fasciculi gracilis** and **cuneatus**, containing first-order sensory neurones) continue rostrally from the spinal cord to their termination in the **nuclei gracilis** and **cuneatus**, whose locations are marked by two small elevations, the gracile and cuneate tubercles.

The caudal two-thirds of the medulla contains the rostral continuation of the central canal of the spinal cord and is, thus, sometimes referred to as the 'closed' portion of the medulla. In passing rostrally, the central canal moves progressively more dorsally until, in the rostral medulla, it opens out into the fourth ventricle. This portion is, thus, sometimes referred to as the 'open' medulla. The floor of the fourth ventricle forms a shallow, rhomboid depression on the dorsal surface of the rostral medulla and the pons. The transition from medulla to pons is not clearly delineated on the dorsal surface of the brain stem but, approximately, the caudal third of the floor of the fourth ventricle constitutes the dorsal aspect of the rostral medulla, whilst the rostral two-thirds of the ventricular floor is made up of the dorsal aspect of the pons. The fourth ventricle is widest at the level of the pontomedullary junction where a **lateral recess** extends to the lateral margin of the

Fig. 6.1 **The dorsal aspect of the brain stem**.

brain stem. At this point the small **lateral aperture** (**foramen of Luschka**) provides passage for cerebrospinal fluid within the fourth ventricle to reach the subarachnoid space surrounding the brain. The lateral walls of the rostral part of the fourth ventricle are made up of the **superior** and **inferior cerebellar peduncles**, connecting the brain stem with the cerebellum. In the rostral pons the walls converge until, at the pontomesencephalic junction, the fourth ventricle becomes continuous with a small channel, the **cerebral aqueduct**, which passes throughout the length of the midbrain.

The dorsal aspect of the midbrain is marked by four paired elevations, the **superior** and **inferior colliculi**, which are parts of the visual and auditory systems, respectively. The **trochlear nerve** (fourth cranial nerve) emerges immediately caudal to the inferior colliculus.

VENTRAL SURFACE OF THE BRAIN STEM
(Figs 6.2 and 6.3)

On the ventral surface of the medulla, prominent longitudinal columns, the **pyramids**, run on either side of the ventral median fissure. The pyramid gives its name to the underlying **pyramidal** or **corticospinal tract** which consists of descending fibres originating from the ipsilateral cerebral cortex. In the caudal medulla

75–90% of these fibres cross over in the **decussation of the pyramids**, partly obscuring the ventral median fissure as they do so, to form the lateral corticospinal tract of the spinal cord. Lateral to the pyramid lies an elongated elevation, the olive, within which lies the **inferior olivary nucleus** which has connections primarily with the cerebellum and, thus, is involved with the control of movement.

The transition from medulla to pons is clearly delineated on the ventral surface. The ventral part of the pons is dominated by a transverse system of fibres (the **transverse pontine fibres** or **pontocerebellar fibres**) which originate from cells in the ventral pons (**pontine nuclei**) and pass through the contralateral **middle cerebellar peduncle**, to enter the cerebellar hemisphere. The pontine nuclei receive corticopontine fibres from the cerebral cortex (including the motor cortex) and constitute an important connection between cerebral and cerebellar cortices, involved in the coordination of movement. The massive system of transverse pontine fibres obscures the underlying corticospinal tract.

The ventral surface of the midbrain consists, on either side, of a massive column of descending fibres, the **crus cerebri** or **basis pedunculi**. In the midline, the two crura cerebri are separated by a depression called the interpeduncular fossa. The crus cerebri is continu-

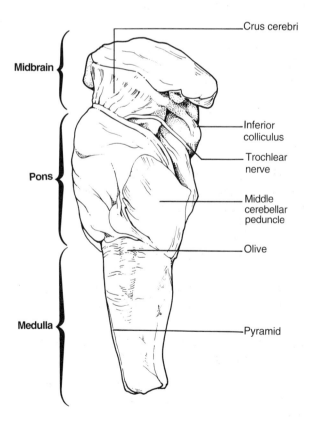

Fig. 6.2 **The ventral aspect of the brain stem**.

Fig. 6.3 **The lateral aspect of the brain stem**.

ous rostrally with the internal capsule of the cerebral hemisphere (see Fig. 1.13) and consists of corticobulbar and corticospinal fibres which have left the cerebral hemisphere via the internal capsule on their way to the brain stem and spinal cord. They are primarily motor in function.

External features of the brain stem

- The brain stem consists of the medulla oblongata, pons and midbrain.
- On the dorsal aspect of the brain stem can be seen the dorsal columns, the floor of the fourth ventricle and the superior and inferior colliculi.
- The dorsal aspect of the rostral medulla and the pons form the floor of the fourth ventricle; the lateral and median apertures of the fourth ventricle permit the passage of cerebrospinal fluid into the subarachnoid space. The cerebral aqueduct runs through the midbrain, beneath the colliculi.
- On the ventral aspect of the brain stem can be seen the pyramids, transverse pontine fibres and the crura cerebri.
- The inferior, middle and superior cerebellar peduncles connect the cerebellum to the medulla, pons and midbrain, respectively.

INTERNAL STRUCTURE OF THE BRAIN STEM

CAUDAL MEDULLA (Fig. 6.4)

At the transition from spinal cord to medulla the pattern of grey and white matter undergoes considerable rearrangement. The ventral horn becomes much attenuated. The dorsal horn is replaced by the caudal part of the **trigeminal sensory nucleus (nucleus of the spinal tract of the trigeminal nerve)**. The trigeminal sensory nucleus is regarded as the brainstem homologue of the dorsal horn since it receives primary afferent fibres conveying general sensation from the head, which enter the brain stem in the trigeminal nerve. It is a large nucleus which extends the whole length of the brain stem and into the upper segments of the spinal cord. This latter, caudal part of the trigeminal nucleus is particularly associated with the modalities of pain and temperature. The trigeminal nerve attaches to the pons and, thus, fibres which terminate in the parts of the trigeminal nucleus caudal to this level descend in a tract (**the spinal tract of the trigeminal**) which lies immediately superficial to the nucleus.

In the ventral medulla the majority of fibres of the pyramid undergo decussation, then pass laterally, dorsally and caudally to form the lateral corticospinal tract.

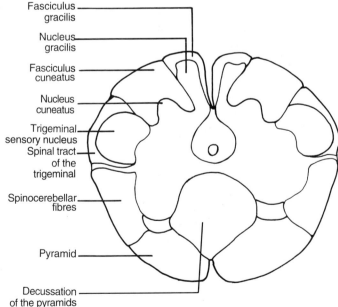

Fasciculus gracilis
Nucleus gracilis
Fasciculus cuneatus
Nucleus cuneatus
Trigeminal sensory nucleus
Spinal tract of the trigeminal
Spinocerebellar fibres
Pyramid
Decussation of the pyramids

Fig. 6.4 **Transverse section through the caudal medulla at the level of the decussation of the pyramids.**
The sections shown in Figs 6.4–6.12 have been stained by the Weigert-Pal method. Areas rich in nerve fibres stain darkly while areas rich in cell bodies are relatively pale.

MID MEDULLA (Fig. 6.5)

On the ventral surface the pyramids are prominent, above their decussation. On the dorsal surface the dorsal columns reach their termination in the gracile and cuneate nuclei which appear beneath their respective tracts. The dorsal columns consist of first-order sensory neurones whose cell bodies lie in the dorsal root ganglia and whose central processes have ascended ipsilaterally through the cord and into the medulla. They terminate in the nucleus gracilis and cuneatus upon the cell bodies of second-order neurones. The axons of these neurones course ventrally and medially as **internal arcuate fibres**, decussating in the midline. Thereafter, they turn rostrally forming a distinct tract, the **medial lemniscus**, which runs through the rostral medulla, the pons and midbrain to terminate in the ventral posterior nucleus of the thalamus.

ROSTRAL MEDULLA (Fig. 6.6)

On the ventral surface of the medulla the pyramids remain conspicuous. Immediately dorsal to the medial aspect of the pyramid lies the medial lemniscus, on either side of the midline. Dorsolateral to the pyramid and lateral to the medial lemniscus is the **inferior olivary nucleus**, lying within the prominence of the olive. The inferior olivary nucleus has the appearance of a crenated bag with an opening, or hilum, facing medially through which afferent and efferent fibres pass. It is concerned with the control of movement. It receives afferents from the motor and sensory cortices of the cerebral hemisphere and from the red nucleus of the midbrain. Its main efferent connection is to the cerebellum via the inferior cerebellar peduncle. Within the cerebellum its axons, known as climbing fibres, end in excitatory synapses in the dentate nucleus and upon Purkinje cells of the cerebellar cortex.

Dorsal to the inferior olivary nucleus and lateral to the medial lemniscus lie second-order sensory fibres ascending to the ventral posterior thalamus from the trigeminal nucleus (the **trigeminothalamic tract**) and from the spinal cord (spinothalamic fibres, referred to in the brain stem as the **spinal lemniscus**).

The dorsal surface of the rostral medulla forms part of the floor of the fourth ventricle. Both immediately and deep beneath the floor of the ventricle lie a number of cranial nerve nuclei, some of which can be clearly

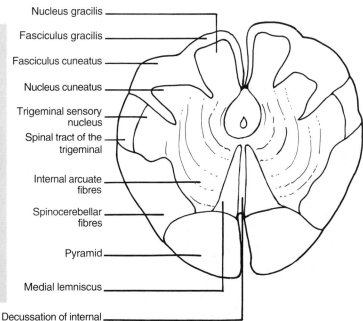

Nucleus gracilis

Fasciculus gracilis

Fasciculus cuneatus

Nucleus cuneatus

Trigeminal sensory nucleus

Spinal tract of the trigeminal

Internal arcuate fibres

Spinocerebellar fibres

Pyramid

Medial lemniscus

Decussation of internal arcuate fibres

Fig. 6.5 **Transverse section through the mid medulla at the level of the sensory decussation.**

identified in simply stained sections, others of which cannot. Immediately beneath the ventricular floor, just lateral to the midline lies the **hypoglossal nucleus** which contains motor neurones innervating the muscles of the tongue via the hypoglossal nerve. Lateral to the hypoglossal nucleus lies the **dorsal (motor) nucleus of the vagus**, containing preganglionic parasympathetic neurones which run in the vagus nerve. The most caudal aspect of the ventricular floor is known as the **area postrema**. At this point the blood–brain barrier, which limits the passage of certain chemicals from the blood to the brain, is absent. This region is the central site of action of substances which cause vomiting (emetics).

In the lateral part of the floor of the fourth ventricle are located the **vestibular nuclei** which receive primary afferent fibres from the vestibular nerve. Ventromedial to the hypoglossal nucleus, close to the midline, is located the **medial longitudinal fasciculus**. This consists of both ascending and descending fibres and can be identified also in the pons and midbrain. Within the brain stem it links the vestibular nuclei with the nuclei supplying the extraocular muscles (abducens, trochlear and oculomotor nuclei) and subserves the coordination of head and eye movements.

The dorsolateral part of the rostral medulla is dominated by the inferior cerebellar peduncle, or **restiform**

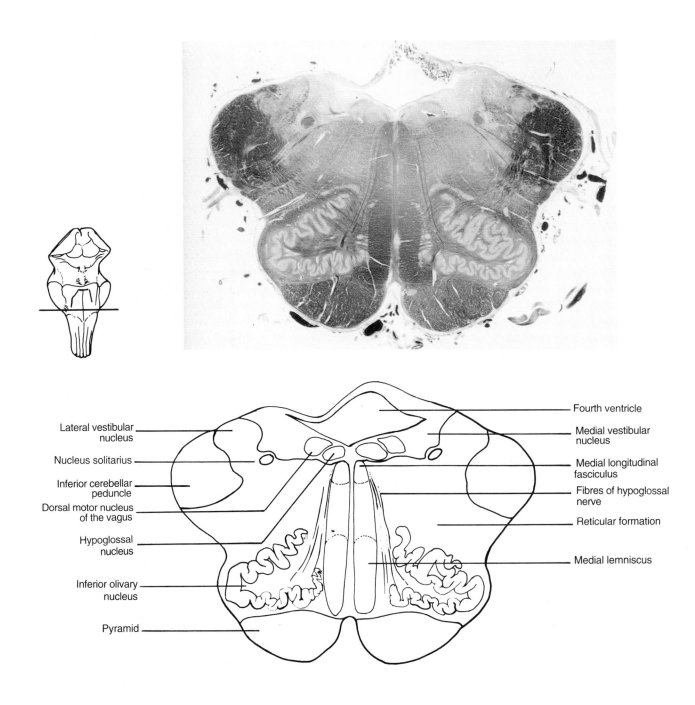

Fig. 6.6 **Transverse section through the rostral medulla at the level of the inferior olivary nucleus**.

body. This consists of fibres passing between the medulla and the cerebellum. Prominent amongst these are olivocerebellar fibres, connections between the vestibular nuclei and the cerebellum, and the fibres of the dorsal spinocerebellar tract, conveying proprioceptive information from the limbs. On the dorsal and lateral aspects of the inferior cerebellar peduncle lie the dorsal and ventral **cochlear nuclei** which receive afferent fibres from the cochlear nerve. Deep beneath the ventricular floor, just dorsal to the inferior olivary nucleus, is located the **nucleus ambiguus**. This sends motor fibres into the glossopharyngeal, vagus and accessory nerves and thence to the muscles of the pharynx and larynx.

PONS (Figs 6.7–6.9)

The pons may be divided into a ventral, or basal, portion and a dorsal portion, also known as the **tegmentum**. The ventral portion is marked by numerous transversely oriented fascicles of pontocerebellar fibres, which originate from scattered cell groups, the **pontine nuclei**, and which pass to the contralateral side of the cerebellum through the massive middle cerebellar peduncle (**brachium pontis**). Corticospinal fibres (which continue into the medullary pyramid) appear as small separate bundles running longitudinally between the fascicles of transverse pontine fibres.

The ascending fibres of the medial lemniscus become separated from the pyramid and displaced dorsally, together with the spinal lemniscus and trigeminothalamic tract, by intervening transverse

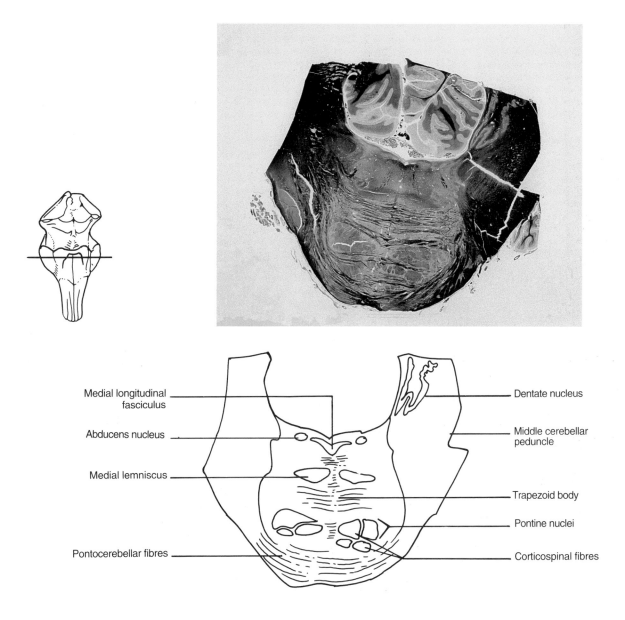

Fig. 6.7 **Transverse section through the caudal pons**.

pontocerebellar fibres. The medial lemniscus also rotates through 90° so that it lies almost horizontally, marking the boundary between ventral and tegmental portions of the pons. In the caudal pons (Fig. 6.7), an additional group of transversely running fibres are found located ventral to the ascending lemniscal fibres but dorsal to the pontocerebellar fibres. This is the **trapezoid body**, which consists of acoustic fibres crossing the brain stem from the cochlear nuclei, to ascend into the midbrain as the **lateral lemniscus** and terminate in the inferior colliculus.

Beneath the floor of the fourth ventricle, in the pontine tegmentum, lie a number of cranial nerve nuclei. These include the **abducens nucleus** (lateral rectus muscle), the **facial motor nucleus** (muscles of facial expression) and the **trigeminal motor nucleus** (muscles of mastication), which each supply motor axons to their respective cranial nerves. Also the trigeminal sensory nucleus, already encountered in the medulla, reaches its maximum extent in the pons, adjacent to the origin of the trigeminal nerve.

In the rostral half of the pons the superior cerebellar peduncles form the lateral walls of the fourth ventricle, the thin superior medullary velum spanning between

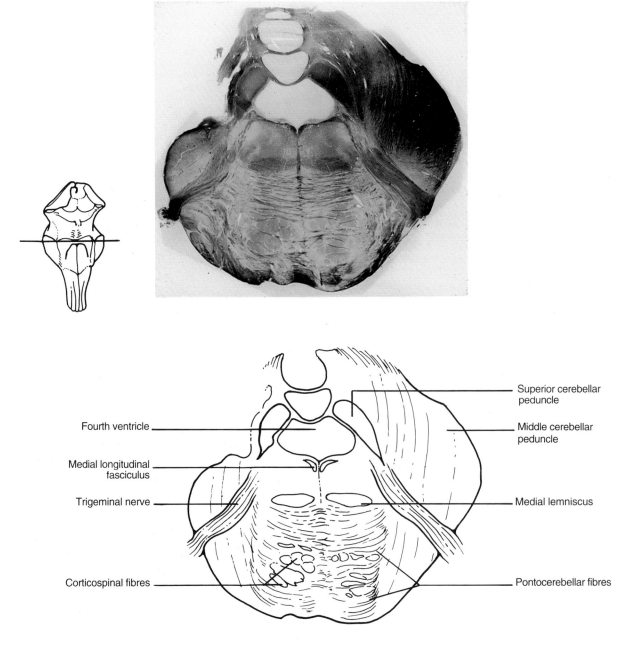

Fig. 6.8 **Transverse section through the mid pons at the level of the trigeminal nerve.**

them to form its roof. The superior peduncle contains some cerebellar afferent fibres, such as the ventral spinocerebellar tract which conveys proprioceptive information from the limbs. It consists mainly, however, of ascending cerebellar efferents, concerned with the coordination of movement, which are destined for the red nucleus of the midbrain and the ventral lateral nucleus of the thalamus. The superior cerebellar peduncles converge towards the midline as they pass into the midbrain.

MIDBRAIN (Figs 6.10–6.12)

The midbrain is formally divided into dorsal and ventral portions at the level of the cerebral aqueduct. The dorsal portion is known as the **tectum** which consists largely of the **inferior** and **superior colliculi (corpora quadrigemina)**. The ventral portion of the midbrain is known as the **tegmentum**. It is bounded ventrally by the massive fibre system of the crus cerebri. The term **cerebral peduncle** is sometimes used as a synonym for crus cerebri, but strictly speaking, the cerebral peduncle refers to the whole midbrain, on either side, excluding the tectum.

In the caudal half of the midbrain, the inferior

Fig. 6.9 **Transverse section through the rostral pons.**

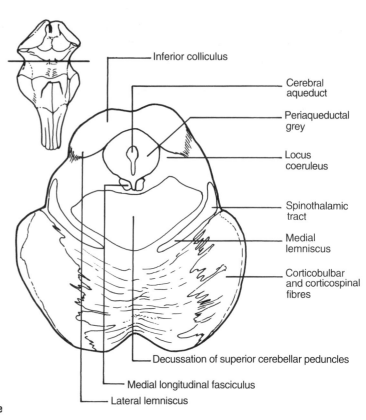

Fig. 6.10 **Transverse section through the brain stem at the level of the pontine-mesencephalic junction**.

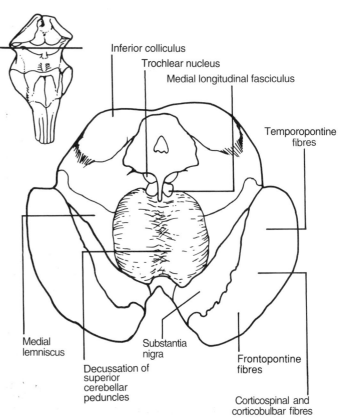

Fig. 6.11 **Transverse section through the caudal midbrain at the level of the inferior colliculus.**

colliculus constitutes part of the **ascending acoustic (auditory) projection**. Ascending auditory fibres run in the lateral lemniscus which terminates in the inferior colliculus. Efferent fibres from the colliculus terminate in the **medial geniculate nucleus** of the thalamus, which in turn projects to the auditory cortex of the temporal lobe.

The superior colliculus of the rostral half of the midbrain is part of the visual system. Its main afferents are corticotectal fibres originating from the visual cortex of the occipital lobe and from the frontal eye field of the frontal lobe. These inputs are concerned with controlling movements of the eyes, such as occur when a moving object is followed (smooth pursuit) or when the direction of the gaze is altered (saccadic eye movements). In addition, corticotectal fibres from the visual cortex are involved in the **accommodation reflex**.

A small number of visual fibres running in the optic tract terminate just rostral to the superior colliculus in the **pretectal nucleus**. This nucleus has connections with parasympathetic neurones controlling the smooth muscle of the eye and is part of the circuit mediating the **pupillary light reflex**.

Ventral to the colliculi the cerebral aqueduct runs the length of the midbrain. Surrounding the aqueduct is a pear-shaped arrangement of grey matter, the **periaqueductal** (or **central**) **grey**. In the ventral part of the periaqueductal grey, at the levels of the inferior and superior colliculi, respectively, lie the **trochlear** and **oculomotor nuclei**, which innervate the extraocular muscles controlling eye movements. Close to the nuclei runs the medial longitudinal fasciculus, which

Fig. 6.12 **Transverse section through the rostral midbrain at the level of the superior colliculus.**

links them to the abducens nucleus in the pons and is important in the control of gaze.

At the level of the inferior colliculus (Figs 6.10 and 6.11), the central portion of the tegmentum is dominated by the superior cerebellar peduncles (**brachium conjunctivum**). These fibres have originated in the cerebellum, coursing ventromedially as they run into the midbrain. Beneath the inferior colliculus the superior cerebellar peduncles decussate in the midline. Rostral to the decussation, at the level of the superior colliculus (Fig. 6.12), the central portion of the tegmentum is occupied by the **red nucleus**, in which some of the fibres of the superior cerebellar peduncle terminate.

The red nucleus is involved in motor control. Its other major source of afferents is the motor cortex of the frontal lobe. Efferent fibres from the red nucleus cross in the ventral tegmental decussation and descend to the spinal cord in the **rubrospinal tract**. In addition, the red nucleus projects to the inferior olivary nucleus of the medulla, via the **central tegmental tract**.

The most ventral part of the midbrain tegmentum is occupied by the **substantia nigra**. A subdivision of this nucleus, known as the **pars compacta**, consists of pigmented, melanin-containing, neurones which synthesise dopamine as their transmitter. These neurones project to the caudate nucleus and putamen of the basal

---

Brain stem lesions

A unilateral brain stem lesion due to stroke, tumour or multiple sclerosis, causes ipsilateral cranial nerve dysfunction, contralateral spastic hemiparesis, hyperreflexia and an extensor plantar response (upper motor neurone lesion), contralateral hemi-sensory loss and ipsilateral incoordination (Fig. 6.13); refer also to Ch. 1 (Fig. 1.26). A bilateral lesion destroys the 'vital centres' for respiration and the circulation, leading to

coma and death. Multiple sclerosis can affect eye movements due to demyelination of the medial longitudinal fasciculus, which interferes with conjugate ocular deviation. Typically, on horizontal gaze, the abducting eye moves normally but the adducting eye fails to follow. Adduction is preserved on convergence. **Internuclear ophthalmoplegia** is the term used to describe this disorder (Fig. 6.14).

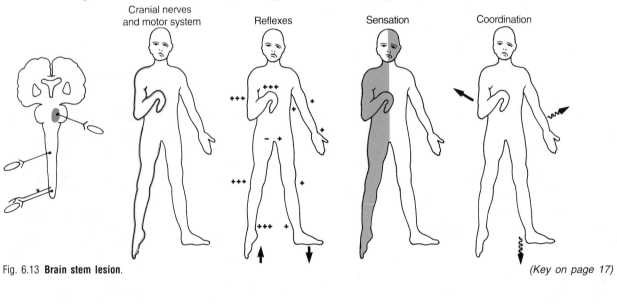

Fig. 6.13 **Brain stem lesion**.   *(Key on page 17)*

Fig. 6.14 **Internuclear ophthalmoplegia**.

ganglia in the forebrain. Degeneration of the substantia nigra, pars compacta, is associated with Parkinson's disease.

Ventral to the substantia nigra lies the massive crus cerebri. This consists entirely of descending cortical efferent fibres which have left the cerebral hemisphere by traversing the internal capsule. Approximately the middle half of the crus consists of **corticobulbar** and **corticospinal fibres**. The corticobulbar fibres end predominantly in or near the motor cranial nerve nuclei of the brain stem. The corticospinal (pyramidal) fibres traverse the pons to enter the medullary pyramid and, thence, the corticospinal tract.

On either side of the corticobulbar and corticospinal fibres, the crus cerebri contains corticopontine fibres which originate from widespread regions of the cerebral cortex and terminate in the pontine nuclei of the ventral pons. From the pontine nuclei connections are established with the cerebellum, via the middle cerebellar peduncle, which are involved in the coordination of movement.

RETICULAR FORMATION

The reticular formation consists of a complex matrix of neurones which extends throughout the length of the brain stem. This is, in phylogenetic terms, a relatively old part of the brain stem and its neurones fulfil a number of important functions, some of which are necessary for survival. The reticular formation has widespread afferent and efferent connections with other parts of the CNS, which reflect its complex and multimodal functions. Some reticular neurones have long axons which ascend and descend for considerable distances within the brain stem, allowing profuse interaction with other neuronal systems. Within the reticular formation a number of individual nuclei are recognised. Some functions are subserved, however, by more dispersed networks which do not correspond exactly to anatomically identified nuclei. The latter applies to the so-called respiratory and cardiovascular centres. These consist of diffuse neuronal networks, located within the medullary and caudal pontine reticular formation, which control respiratory movements and cardiovascular function.

Descending **reticulospinal tracts** originate from the medullary and pontine reticular formation (Chapter 5). These predominantly influence muscle tone and posture. Some of the ascending fibres of the reticular formation constitute the **reticular activating system**. These neurones receive input, either directly or indirectly, from multiple sensory sources. Through the

intermediary of thalamic nuclei, they cause activation of the cerebral cortex and heightened arousal.

The **raphe nuclei** are a group of midline nuclei which extend throughout the length of the brain stem. Many of the neurones of these nuclei are serotonergic (that is to say, utilise serotonin or 5-hydroxytryptamine as their transmitter). Their axons are widely distributed throughout the CNS. In particular, ascending fibres to forebrain structures are involved in the neural mechanisms of sleep and descending fibres to the spinal cord are involved in the modulation of nociceptive mechanisms.

The **locus coeruleus** is a group of pigmented neurones which lies in the brain stem tegmentum of the caudal midbrain and rostral pons. It is the principal noradrenergic cell group of the brain. It projects to many areas of the CNS. Ascending fibres project to the cerebellum, hypothalamus, thalamus, limbic structures and cerebral cortex. Descending fibres project widely throughout the brain stem and spinal cord. The locus coeruleus, like the raphe nuclei, has been implicated in the neural mechanisms regulating sleep, particularly REM (rapid eye movement) sleep.

Internal structure of the brain stem

- Cranial nerves III–XII attach to the brain stem, their fibres either originating from, or terminating in, the cranial nerve nuclei.
- The reticular formation controls the level of consciousness, the cardiovascular system and the respiratory system.
- Ascending sensory systems pass through the brain stem en route to the thalamus. First-order proprioceptive fibres in the dorsal columns relay in the dorsal column nuclei. Second-order fibres decussate to form the medial lemniscus. Spinothalamic fibres form the spinal lemniscus.
- Descending fibre systems both pass through the brain stem and originate within it.
- The corticospinal tract runs through the crus cerebri, the basal part of the pons and the medullary pyramid; 75–90% of fibres cross in the pyramidal decussation to form the lateral corticospinal tract.
- The reticular formation, red nucleus and vestibular nuclei give rise to descending fibres which pass to the spinal cord.

Cranial nerves and cranial nerve nuclei

There are twelve, bilaterally paired, cranial nerves which carry afferent and efferent fibres between the brain and peripheral structures, principally of the head and neck. They are individually named and numbered (Roman numerals) according to the rostrocaudal sequence in which they attach to the brain (Fig. 7.1):

I	olfactory	VII	facial
II	optic	VIII	vestibulocochlear
III	oculomotor	IX	glossopharyngeal
IV	trochlear	X	vagus
V	trigeminal	XI	accessory
VI	abducens	XII	hypoglossal

Fig. 7.1 **The base of the brain illustrating the locations of the cranial nerves**. The points of attachment are shown, except for the trochlear nerve which arises from the dorsal aspect of the brain stem.

The first two cranial nerves attach directly to the forebrain, whilst the rest attach to the brain stem. The olfactory system is closely associated, both structurally and functionally, with parts of the forebrain collectively referred to as the limbic system and these are considered together in Chapter 13. The visual system is described in Chapter 12. Cranial nerves III–XII are associated with various nuclei within the brain stem, the cranial nerve nuclei, which either receive cranial nerve afferents or contain the cell bodies of efferent neurones whose axons leave the brain in cranial nerves. The locations of these nuclei are illustrated in Fig. 7.2.

AFFERENT CRANIAL NERVE NUCLEI

Fibres carrying common sensation (touch, pressure, pain, temperature), entering the brain predominantly in the trigeminal nerve at the level of the pons, terminate in the **trigeminal sensory nucleus**. This is a large nucleus which extends the whole length of the brain stem and into the cervical spinal cord. Fibres conveying the special senses of hearing and motion\ positional sense run in the vestibulocochlear nerve. They terminate in the **vestibular** and **cochlear nuclei**, respectively, which are located in the medulla, in and near to the lateral part of the floor of the fourth ventricle. Visceral afferents, including taste fibres, terminate in the **nucleus solitarius** of the medulla.

EFFERENT CRANIAL NERVE NUCLEI

On the basis of their embryological derivation, the efferent cranial nerve nuclei can be divided into three groups, each lying in a discontinuous longitudinal column.

Nuclei of the somatic efferent cell column

The somatic efferent cell column lies near to the midline and consists of the nuclei of the III, IV, VI, and XII nerves. The **oculomotor nucleus** lies in the ventral apex of the periaqueductal grey of the midbrain, at the

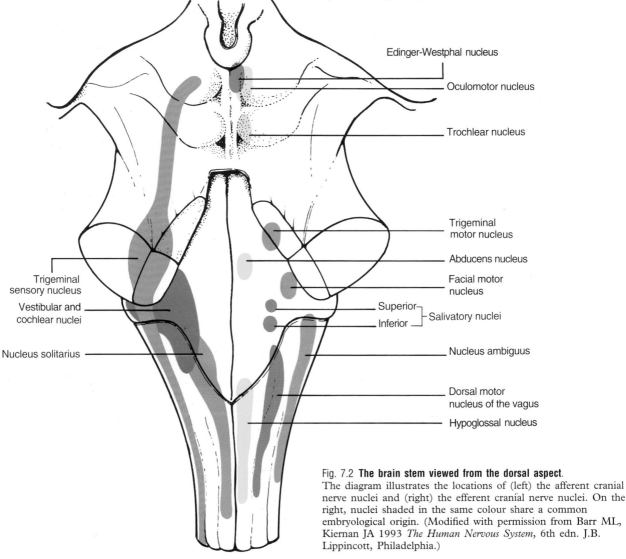

Edinger-Westphal nucleus
Oculomotor nucleus
Trochlear nucleus
Trigeminal motor nucleus
Abducens nucleus
Facial motor nucleus
Superior ⌉
Inferior ⌋ Salivatory nuclei
Nucleus ambiguus
Dorsal motor nucleus of the vagus
Hypoglossal nucleus

Trigeminal sensory nucleus
Vestibular and cochlear nuclei
Nucleus solitarius

Fig. 7.2 **The brain stem viewed from the dorsal aspect**.
The diagram illustrates the locations of (left) the afferent cranial nerve nuclei and (right) the efferent cranial nerve nuclei. On the right, nuclei shaded in the same colour share a common embryological origin. (Modified with permission from Barr ML, Kiernan JA 1993 *The Human Nervous System*, 6th edn. J.B. Lippincott, Philadelphia.)

level of the superior colliculus. Its efferent fibres run in the oculomotor nerve to innervate the levator palpebrae superioris and all of the extraocular muscles, except the superior oblique and lateral rectus. The **trochlear nucleus** also lies in the midbrain, at the ventral border of the periaqueductal grey, but at the level of the inferior colliculus. Fibres leave in the trochlear nerve to innervate the superior oblique muscle of the eye. The **abducens nucleus** is located in the caudal pons beneath the floor of the fourth ventricle. Its efferents run in the abducens nerve and innervate the lateral rectus muscle. In the medulla lies the **hypoglossal nucleus**, which innervates the intrinsic and extrinsic muscles of the tongue via the hypoglossal nerve.

Nuclei of the branchiomotor cell column

The branchiomotor cell column innervates striated muscles derived from the branchial arches. In the tegmentum of the mid-pons is located the **trigeminal motor nucleus** which supplies fibres to the trigeminal nerve and innervates the muscles of mastication, tensor tympani, tensor veli palitini, mylohyoid and the anterior belly of the digastric muscle. In the caudal pontine tegmentum lies the **facial motor nucleus**. This innervates the muscles of facial expression and the stapedius muscle via the facial nerve. Within the medulla lies the **nucleus ambiguus**. This long nucleus sends motor fibres in the glossopharyngeal, vagus and cranial part of the accessory nerve to innervate muscles of the pharynx and larynx.

Nuclei of the parasympathetic cell column

The parasympathetic cell column consists of preganglionic parasympathetic neurones which send axons into the III, VII, IX and X cranial nerves. The most rostral cell group constitutes the **Edinger–Westphal nucleus** which lies in the midbrain periaqueductal

grey, adjacent to the oculomotor nucleus. Its axons leave in the oculomotor nerve and pass to the ciliary ganglion, from which postganglionic fibres innervate the sphincter pupillae and ciliary muscle of the eye. In the pontine tegmentum lie two cell groups, the **superior** and **inferior salivatory nuclei**. The superior salivatory nucleus supplies preganglionic fibres to the facial nerve which terminate in the pterygopalatine and submandibular ganglia. Postganglionic fibres from the pterygopalatine ganglion innervate the lacrimal gland and the nasal and oral mucous membranes. Those from the submandibular ganglion innervate the submandibular and sublingual salivary glands. The inferior salivatory nucleus sends preganglionic fibres into the glossopharyngeal nerve. These terminate in the otic ganglion which in turn sends postganglionic axons to the parotid salivary gland. The largest preganglionic parasympathetic cell group lies in the medulla and constitutes the **dorsal motor nucleus of the vagus**. Its rostral portion lies immediately beneath the floor of the fourth ventricle, lateral to the hypoglossal nucleus. Fibres leave in the vagus nerve and are widely distributed to thoracic and abdominal viscera.

CRANIAL NERVES

III: OCULOMOTOR NERVE

The oculomotor nerve contains somatic motor neurones which innervate extraocular muscles and preganglionic parasympathetic neurones which, via the intermediary of the ciliary ganglion, control the smooth muscle within the eye.

The motor neurones serving the extraocular muscles have their cell bodies in the **oculomotor nucleus** which lies at the base of the periaqueductal grey of the midbrain at the level of the superior colliculus (Fig. 7.3). Preganglionic parasympathetic neurones arise from

Fig. 7.3 **Transverse section through the midbrain at the level of the superior colliculus.**
The diagram shows the origin and course of oculomotor nerve fibres within the brain stem.

Superior colliculus

Cerebral aqueduct

Oculomotor nucleus

Red nucleus

Crus cerebri

Periaqueductal grey

Edinger-Westphal nucleus

Medial longitudinal fasciculus

Substantia nigra

Oculomotor nerve

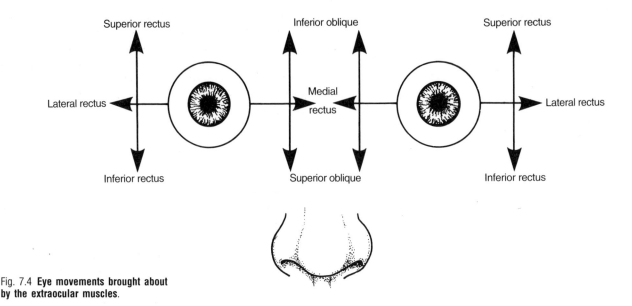

Fig. 7.4 **Eye movements brought about by the extraocular muscles**.

the nearby Edinger–Westphal nucleus. Fibres from both sources course ventrally through the midbrain tegmentum, many of them traversing the red nucleus, to exit on the medial aspect of the crus cerebri, within the interpeduncular fossa. The oculomotor nerve passes between the posterior cerebral and superior cerebellar arteries, then runs anteriorly, lying in the wall of the cavernous sinus, before gaining access to the orbit through the superior orbital fissure. The oculomotor nerve supplies all of the extraocular muscles, with the exception of the superior oblique and lateral rectus, and thus functions to elevate, depress and adduct the eyeball (Fig. 7.4). It also innervates the striated muscle of the levator palpebrae superioris. Preganglionic parasympathetic neurones terminate in the ciliary ganglion. From here postganglionic neurones run in the **short ciliary nerves** to innervate the sphincter (constrictor) pupillae muscle of the iris and the ciliary muscle contained within the ciliary body.

Pupillary light reflex

The amount of light entering the eye is regulated by the size of the pupil. Illumination of the retina causes constriction of the pupil, due to contraction of the sphincter pupillae muscle of the iris, thus reducing the amount of light reaching the retina. This is known as the **direct light reflex** (Fig. 7.5). Even if only one retina is illuminated (e.g. during clinical examination) the pupils of both eyes constrict. The constriction of the pupil of the non-illuminated eye is called the **consensual light reflex**. The afferent limb of the light reflex consists of a small contingent of optic tract fibres which pass directly from the eye to the **pretectal area**, just rostral to the superior colliculus, rather than the lateral geniculate nucleus of the thalamus (see also Ch. 12). Neurones of the pretectal area project bilaterally

to the Edinger–Westphal nuclei whose efferent fibres leave in the oculomotor nerve.

Accommodation reflex

Fixation upon a nearby object by convergence of the optic axes involves concomitant contraction of the ciliary muscle to increase the convexity of the lens, thus focusing the image. It is also accompanied by pupillary constriction. The phenomenon involves the visual cortex, with corticobulbar fibres activating the parasympathetic neurones of the Edinger–Westphal nuclei bilaterally.

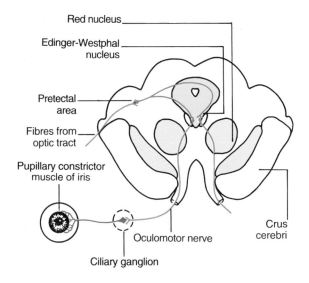

Fig. 7.5 **Schematic representation of a transverse section through the most rostral part of the midbrain.**
The diagram shows the pathways involved in the pupillary light reflex.

IV: TROCHLEAR NERVE

The trochlear nerve contains only somatic motor neurones. These arise in the **trochlear nucleus**, which lies in the midbrain periaqueductal grey at the level of the inferior colliculus (Fig. 7.6). Axons pass dorsally, around the periaqueductal grey, and cross the midline. The trochlear nerve emerges from the dorsal aspect of the brain stem (the only cranial nerve to do so) just caudal to the inferior colliculus. The nerve courses round the cerebral peduncle to gain the ventral aspect

of the brain, passing between the posterior cerebral and superior cerebellar arteries, as does the oculomotor nerve. It then runs anteriorly, lying in the lateral wall of the cavernous sinus, entering the orbit through the superior orbital fissure. It supplies just one muscle, the **superior oblique**, which moves the eyeball downwards and medially.

VI: ABDUCENS NERVE

The abducens, like the trochlear nerve, contains only somatic motor neurones. The cell bodies of origin are located in the **abducens nucleus**, which lies beneath the floor of the fourth ventricle in the caudal pons (Fig. 7.7). Fibres pass ventrally through the pons and emerge from the ventral surface of the brain stem at the junction between the pons and the pyramid of the medulla. The nerve then passes anteriorly, through the cavernous sinus, enters the orbit through the superior orbital fissure and supplies the lateral rectus muscle, which abducts the eye.

V: TRIGEMINAL NERVE

The trigeminal nerve has both sensory and motor components. It is the main sensory nerve for the head and, additionally, innervates the muscles of mastication. It attaches to the brain stem as two adjacent roots (a large sensory and a smaller motor) on the ventrolateral aspect of the pons, where this merges with the middle cerebellar peduncle (Fig. 7.1).

The sensory fibres of the trigeminal nerve are primary (first-order) sensory neurones whose peripheral processes are distributed via ophthalmic, maxillary and mandibular divisions of the trigeminal to numerous structures of the head (Fig. 7.8). Sensations of touch,

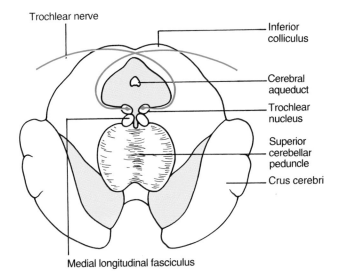

Fig. 7.6 **Transverse section through the midbrain at the level of the inferior colliculus**.
The diagram shows the location of the trochlear nucleus and the course of trochlear nerve fibres.

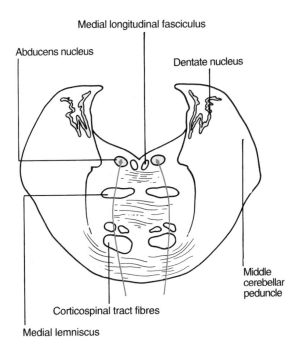

Fig. 7.7 **Transverse section through the caudal pons**.
The diagram shows the location of the abducens nucleus and the course of abducens nerve fibres.

Fig. 7.8 **Superficial distribution of sensory fibres in the three divisions of the trigeminal nerve**.

Lesions of the third, fourth and sixth cranial nerves

A third cranial nerve palsy (Fig. 7.9), due to a lesion of the oculomotor nucleus within the midbrain, or to compression of the peripheral course of the third nerve caused by an aneurysm or tumour, leads to drooping of the eyelid (ptosis), dilation of the pupil, which is unresponsive to light and accommodation, and an inability to move the eyeball upwards, downwards and inwards (adduction).

A sixth cranial nerve palsy (Fig. 7.10), due to a lesion of the abducens nucleus in the pons or to compression of the peripheral course of the nerve by an aneurysm or tumour, leads to an inability to move the eye outwards (abduction).

Combined unilateral palsies of the third, fourth and sixth cranial nerves occur due to lesions along their peripheral course where the nerves run adjacent to each other, such as within the cavernous sinus, at the entrance to the orbit (superior orbital fissure) and within the orbit. There they are vulnerable to compression by tumours and aneurysms. The effects of such unilateral lesions are:

- ptosis
- dilation of the pupil, which is unresponsive to light or accommodation
- paralysis of all eye movements.

Fig. 7.9 **Right oculomotor (III) nerve palsy.** The upper part of the diagram shows ptosis on the right. The lower part shows that, with elevation of the eyelid, the eyeball can be seen to be abducted and the pupil dilated.

Fig. 7.10 **Left abducens (VI) nerve palsy.** On looking in the direction of the arrow, the left eye fails to abduct.

pressure, pain and temperature are relayed from the face and scalp, the cornea, the nasal and oral cavities, including the teeth and gums, and the cranial dura mater. In addition, proprioceptive fibres are carried from the muscles of mastication and the temporomandibular joint. The cell bodies of afferents in the trigeminal nerve, with the exception of those conveying proprioception, are located in the **trigeminal** (or **semilunar**) **ganglion** located at the convergence of the ophthalmic, maxillary and mandibular nerves. The central processes of these cells terminate in the **trigeminal sensory nucleus** (Fig. 7.11).

The trigeminal sensory nucleus is a large structure,

extending throughout the length of the brain stem and into the upper cervical cord. It is considered to consist of three subnuclei. The chief (or principal) sensory nucleus lies in the pontine tegmentum close to the entry of the trigeminal nerve. The **mesencephalic nucleus** extends rostrally into the midbrain. The **spinal nucleus** (or nucleus of the spinal tract of the trigeminal) extends caudally through the medulla and into the cord where it becomes continuous with the substantia gelatinosa, of which it is considered to be the brainstem homologue.

There is a segregated distribution of afferent fibre termination in the trigeminal nucleus. Fibres convey-

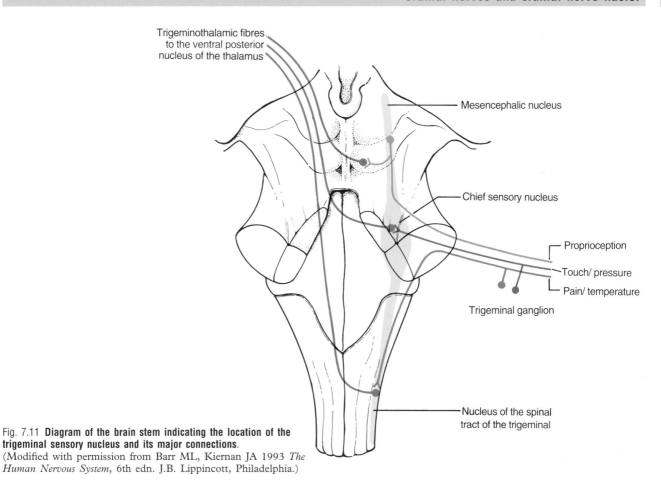

Trigeminothalamic fibres to the ventral posterior nucleus of the thalamus

Mesencephalic nucleus

Chief sensory nucleus

Proprioception

Touch/ pressure

Pain/ temperature

Trigeminal ganglion

Nucleus of the spinal tract of the trigeminal

Fig. 7.11 **Diagram of the brain stem indicating the location of the trigeminal sensory nucleus and its major connections.** (Modified with permission from Barr ML, Kiernan JA 1993 *The Human Nervous System*, 6th edn. J.B. Lippincott, Philadelphia.)

ing touch and pressure terminate in the principal nucleus. Those carrying pain and temperature end in the spinal nucleus, reaching their termination by descending in the spinal tract of the trigeminal which lies immediately superficial to the nucleus. In the upper cervical cord the spinal tract of the trigeminal becomes continuous with Lissauer's tract which carries functionally homologous afferents of spinal nerve origin, prior to their termination in the dorsal horn. Proprioceptive afferents from the muscles of mastica-

tion and the temporomandibular joint have their cell bodies not in the trigeminal ganglion, as might be expected, but in the mesencephalic nucleus of the trigeminal. They are the only primary afferents to have their cell bodies located within the central nervous system. Axons arising from second-order neurones in the trigeminal nucleus decussate to form the contralateral **trigeminothalamic tract** (**trigeminal lemniscus**). This terminates in the contralateral ventral posterior nucleus of the thalamus, which in turn sends fibres to the sensory cortex of the parietal lobe. In addition, the trigeminal nucleus sends fibres to the cerebellum and establishes reflex connections with certain motor cell groups of the brain stem. Prominent amongst these is the facial nucleus, through which are mediated facial grimacing and eye closure (corneal reflex) in response to noxious stimulation in the territory served by the trigeminal.

The motor axons of the trigeminal nerve arise from cells in the trigeminal motor nucleus which lies in the pontine tegmentum medial to the principal sensory nucleus. Axons leave the pons in the motor root of the trigeminal and then join the mandibular division. They innervate various muscles, the most significant of which are the muscles of mastication (masseter and temporalis which close the jaw, and the lateral and medial pterygoids which open the jaw).

Lesions of the trigeminal nerve

Herpes zoster infection of the sensory roots of the trigeminal nerve (**shingles**) leads to pain and the eruption of vesicles localised to the dermatome supplied by one or other of the ophthalmic, maxillary and mandibular branches of the trigeminal nerve.

In **syringobulbia**, central cavitation of the medulla caudal to the fourth ventricle leads to preferential compressive destruction of decussating trigeminothalamic fibres, causing selective loss of pain and temperature sensibility (dissociated sensory loss) in the face (cf. syringomyelia).

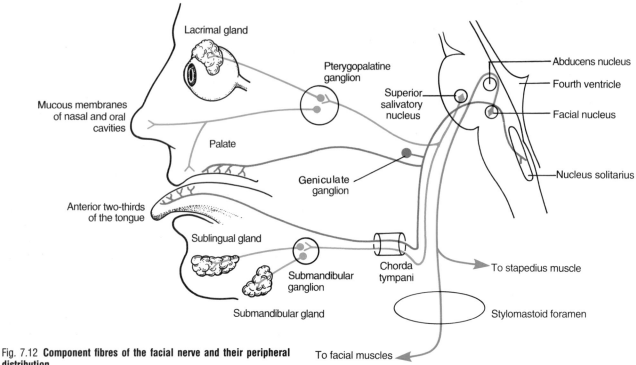

Fig. 7.12 **Component fibres of the facial nerve and their peripheral distribution**.
(Red=motor, green=sensory, blue=parasympathetic.)

VII: FACIAL NERVE

The facial nerve contains sensory, motor and parasympathetic components (Fig. 7.12). It joins the brain stem at the ventrolateral aspect of the caudal pons, near the pontomedullary junction, in a region known as the **cerebellopontine angle**. The nerve consists of two roots, the more lateral (sometimes called the nervus intermedius) containing sensory and parasympathetic fibres, the more medial root being composed of motor axons.

The sensory fibres of the facial nerve supply taste sensation from the anterior two-thirds of the tongue, the floor of the mouth and palate and also cutaneous sensation from part of the external ear. The cell bodies of primary afferent neurones lie in the **geniculate ganglion** within the facial canal of the petrous temporal bone. The central processes of taste fibres terminate in the rostral part of the nucleus solitarius of the medulla. Ascending fibres from the nucleus solitarius project to the ventral posterior nucleus of the thalamus, which in turn sends fibres to the sensory cortex of the parietal lobe. Fibres carrying cutaneous sensation terminate in the trigeminal nucleus.

Motor fibres of the facial nerve originate in the facial motor nucleus of the caudal pontine tegmentum (Fig. 7.13). The axons initially pass dorsally, looping over the abducens nucleus beneath the floor of the fourth ventricle, before leaving the brain stem in the motor root of the facial nerve. Motor fibres are distri-

buted to the muscles of facial expression, platysma, stylohyoid, the posterior belly of the digastric muscle and the stapedius muscle of the middle ear.

The facial motor nucleus receives afferents from other brain stem areas for the mediation of certain reflexes and also from the cerebral cortex. Reflex connections are established, which mediate protective eye closure in response to visual stimuli or tactile stimulation of

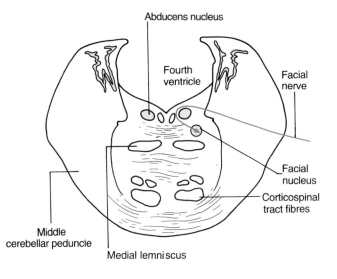

Fig. 7.13 **Transverse section through the pons**.
The diagram shows the origin and course of the motor fibres of the facial nerve.

Bell's palsy

Bell's palsy represents an acute unilateral inflammatory lesion of the facial nerve within its course through the skull. Pain is experienced around the ear and there is paralysis of the facial muscles unilaterally with failure to close the eye, an absent corneal reflex, hyperacusis on the affected side and loss of taste sensation in the anterior two-thirds of the tongue. When the herpes zoster virus is the inflammatory agent, a vesicular rash is apparent in the external auditory canal and the mucous membrane of the oropharynx (**Ramsay Hunt syndrome**).

---

the cornea (**corneal reflex**), by fibres from the superior colliculus and trigeminal sensory nucleus, respectively. In addition, fibres from the superior olivary nucleus, a part of the central auditory pathway, subserve reflex contraction of the stapedius muscle in response to loud noise.

Corticobulbar fibres from motor cortical areas innervate the facial motor nucleus. Those controlling motor neurones which supply the muscles of the upper face (frontalis, orbicularis oculi) are distributed bilaterally. Those which control the motor neurones supplying the muscles of the lower face are entirely crossed. Unilateral upper motor neurone lesions, therefore, give rise to paralysis of the lower facial muscles.

Preganglionic parasympathetic fibres of the facial nerve originate in the superior salivatory nucleus of the pons. Fibres leave the brain stem in the sensory root of the facial nerve (nervus intermedius). From here they pass to parasympathetic ganglia, the submandibular and pterygopalatine ganglia, where they synapse with postganglionic neurones. Those from the submandibular ganglion innervate the submandibular and sublingual salivary glands. Postganglionic fibres from the pterygopalatine ganglion innervate the lacrimal gland and the nasal and oral mucous membranes.

VIII: VESTIBULOCOCHLEAR NERVE

The vestibulocochlear nerve is a sensory nerve which conveys impulses from the inner ear. It has two component parts: the **vestibular nerve** which carries information related to position and movement of the head, and the **cochlear nerve** which carries auditory information. Both divisions contain the axons of first-order sensory neurones whose dendrites make contact with hair cells of either the vestibular or auditory apparatus of the inner ear. Both divisions pass together through the internal auditory meatus (which also contains the facial nerve) and attach to the brain stem at the junction of the medulla and pons, in the region known as the cerebellopontine angle.

The vestibular nerve

The vestibular nerve consists of fibres whose dendrites contact **hair cells** of the vestibular portions of the membranous labyrinth and whose cell bodies are located in the vestibular ganglion, within the internal auditory meatus. The central processes of vestibular fibres mostly end in the **vestibular nuclei** of the rostral medulla. There are four such nuclei (superior, inferior, medial and lateral vestibular nuclei) located close together beneath the lateral part of the floor of the fourth ventricle.

The vestibular nuclei establish contact with a number of other regions for the control of posture, maintenance of equilibrium, coordination of head and eye movements and the conscious awareness of vestibular stimulation. Fibres from the **lateral vestibular (Deiters') nucleus** descend ipsilaterally in the lateral vestibulospinal tract. The vestibular nuclei also contribute fibres to the **medial longitudinal fasciculus (MLF)**, which extends throughout the brain stem and into the spinal cord. The descending component of the MLF is also known as the medial vestibulospinal tract. Vestibulospinal fibres influence the activity of spinal motor neurones concerned with the control of body posture and balance. The ascending part of the medial longitudinal fasciculus establishes connections with the nuclei of the abducens, trochlear and oculomotor nerves for the coordination of head and eye movements. Some efferent fibres from the vestibular nuclei pass through the inferior cerebellar peduncle to the flocculonodular lobe of the cerebellum, which is concerned with the control of equilibrium. Other fibres ascend to the contralateral thalamus (ventral posterior nucleus) which in turn projects to the cerebral cortex. The cortical region responsible for conscious awareness of vestibular sensation is uncertain, but is probably adjacent to the 'head' area of the sensory cortex in the parietal lobe or adjacent to the auditory cortex in the temporal lobe.

The cochlear nerve

The cochlear nerve consists of fibres whose dendrites contact hair cells of the **organ of Corti** within the cochlear duct of the inner ear. The cell bodies of these neurones lie within the cochlea and are collectively called the spiral ganglion. The cochlear nerve joins the brain stem at the level of the rostral medulla. Its fibres bifurcate and end in the **dorsal** and **ventral cochlear nuclei** which lie close to the inferior cerebellar peduncle. From here, the ascending auditory pathway to the thalamus and cerebral cortex (Fig. 7.14) is somewhat more complicated and variable than that for the general senses.

There are several locations, between the medulla and thalamus, where axons may synapse and not all fibres in the pathway behave in the same manner. From

Fig. 7.14 **Principal ascending connections
of the auditory component
of the vestibulocochlear nerve**.

Cerebral hemisphere

Lateral fissure

Superior temporal
gyrus

Medial geniculate nucleus

Red nucleus

**Rostral
midbrain**

Inferior colliculus

**Caudal
midbrain**

Superior cerebellar
peduncle

Nucleus of lateral lemniscus

Lateral lemniscus

Pons

Superior olivary nucleus

Trapezoid body

Ventral cochlear nucleus

Dorsal cochlear nucleus

Cochlear nerve

Medulla

Inferior cerebellar peduncle

Cochlea

Inferior olivary nucleus

Pyramid

the cochlear nuclei, second-order neurones ascend into the pons, some of them crossing to the other side of the pontine tegmentum as the **trapezoid body**. At this level, some fibres may terminate in the **superior olivary nucleus**. This nucleus is the site of origin of olivocochlear fibres, which leave the brain stem in the vestibulocochlear nerve and end in the organ of Corti. They have an inhibitory function and serve to modulate transmission of auditory information to the cochlear nerve. From the superior olivary nuclei, ascending fibres constitute the **lateral lemniscus** which runs through the pontine tegmentum to end in the **inferior colliculus** of the midbrain. Some axons within the lateral lemniscus terminate in a small pontine nucleus called the nucleus of the lateral lemniscus. The superior olivary nucleus and the nucleus of the lateral lemniscus are thought to establish reflex connections with motor neurones of the trigeminal and facial motor nuclei, mediating contraction of the tensor tympani and stapedius muscles in response to loud noise. The inferior colliculus in turn sends axons to the **medial geniculate nucleus** of the thalamus. The final step in the ascending auditory pathway consists of axons which originate in the medial geniculate nucleus and pass through the internal capsule to the **primary auditory cortex** of the temporal lobe. This is located predominantly in **Heschl's gyri**, which are located on the dorsal surface of the **superior temporal gyrus** and, thus, largely hidden within the lateral fissure. Throughout the ascending auditory projection there exists a so-called 'tonotopical' representation of the cochlea, which is analogous to the 'somatotopic' organisation of the pathways for general sensation. Within the brain stem, some ascending fibres decussate whilst others do not. The representation of the cochlea is, therefore, essentially bilateral at all levels rostral to the cochlear nuclei. The region of the temporal lobe surrounding the primary auditory cortex is known as the **auditory association cortex** or **Wernicke's area**. It is here that auditory information is interpreted and given contextual significance. Wernicke's area is important in the processing of language by the brain (p. 112).

Acoustic neuroma

An acoustic neuroma is a benign tumour of the eighth cranial nerve and leads to compression of the nerve and adjacent structures in the **cerebellopontine angle**. Attacks of dizziness accompanied by profound deafness occur and, with expansion of the tumour, ataxia and paralysis of the cranial nerves (especially V–VII) and the limbs. Unilateral and bilateral acoustic neuromas occur in the inherited disease of **neurofibromatosis** in which tumours of the peripheral nerves and skin (neurilemmoma and neurofibroma) can cause cosmetic blemish and deformity.

IX: GLOSSOPHARYNGEAL NERVE

The glossopharyngeal nerve is principally a sensory nerve, although it also contains preganglionic parasympathetic and a few motor fibres. It attaches to the brain stem as a linear series of small rootlets, lateral to the olive in the rostral medulla.

The afferent fibres of the glossopharyngeal nerve convey information from:

- receptors for general sensation in the pharynx, the posterior third of the tongue, eustachian tube and middle ear
- taste buds of the pharynx and the posterior third of the tongue
- chemoreceptors in the carotid body and baroreceptors in the carotid sinus.

Within the brain stem, afferent fibres for general sensation end in the trigeminal sensory nucleus. Fibres carrying touch information from the pharynx and back of the tongue are important for mediating the **gag reflex**, through connections with the nucleus ambiguus and the hypoglossal nucleus. Visceral and taste fibres of the glossopharyngeal nerve terminate in the nucleus solitarius of the medulla.

The motor component of the glossopharyngeal nerve is very small. It arises from cells in the rostral part of the nucleus ambiguus of the medulla and innervates just one muscle, stylopharyngeus, which is involved in swallowing.

Preganglionic parasympathetic fibres in the glossopharyngeal nerve originate in the inferior salivatory nucleus of the rostral medulla. These synapse with postganglionic neurones in the otic ganglion, which in turn innervate the parotid salivary gland.

X: VAGUS NERVE

Rootlets of the vagus nerve attach to the lateral aspect of the medulla, immediately caudal to the glossopharyngeal nerve. It contains afferent, motor and parasympathetic fibres.

The afferent fibres of the vagus convey information from:

- receptors for general sensation in: the pharynx, larynx, oesophagus, tympanic membrane, external auditory meatus and part of the concha of the external ear
- chemoreceptors in the aortic bodies and baroreceptors in the aortic arch
- receptors widely distributed throughout the thoracic and abdominal viscera.

Within the brain stem, receptors for general sensation end in the trigeminal sensory nucleus, whilst visceral afferents end in the nucleus solitarius.

The motor fibres of the vagus (Fig. 7.15) arise from the nucleus ambiguus of the medulla. They innervate

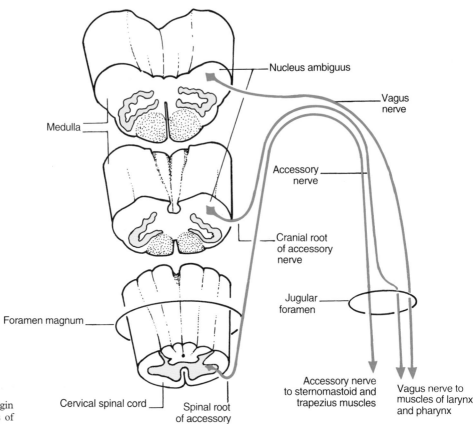

Fig. 7.15 **Diagram of the caudal medulla and rostral spinal cord**. The diagram illustrates the origin and course of the motor fibres of the vagus and accessory nerves.

the muscles of the soft palate, pharynx, larynx and upper part of the oesophagus. The nucleus ambiguus is, thus, crucially important in the control of speech and swallowing. By convention, the most caudal efferents from the nucleus ambiguus are regarded as leaving the brain stem in the cranial roots of the accessory nerve, but these transfer to the vagus nerve proper at the level of the jugular foramen (Fig. 7.15).

The parasympathetic fibres of the vagus nerve originate from the dorsal motor nucleus of the vagus which lies in the medulla, immediately beneath the floor of the fourth ventricle. They are distributed widely throughout the cardiovascular, respiratory and gastrointestinal systems.

XI: ACCESSORY NERVE

The accessory nerve is purely motor in function. It consists of two parts: cranial and spinal. The cranial part emerges from the lateral aspect of the medulla as a linear series of rootlets, which lie immediately caudal to the rootlets of the vagus nerve (Fig. 7.15). The cranial root of the accessory nerve carries fibres which have their origin in the caudal part of the nucleus ambiguus of the medulla. At the level of the jugular foramen these fibres join the vagus nerve and are distributed with it to the muscles of the soft palate, pharynx and larynx.

The spinal root of the accessory nerve arises from motor neurones located in the ventral horn of the spinal grey matter at levels C1–C5 (Fig. 7.15). The axons leave the cord, not through the ventral roots of spinal nerves, but via a series of rootlets which emerge from the lateral aspect of the cord, midway between the dorsal and ventral roots. These rootlets course rostrally, coalescing as they do so, and enter the cranial cavity through the foramen magnum. At the side of the medulla, the spinal root of the accessory nerve briefly joins the cranial root, but the component fibres separate once again as the nerve leaves the cranial cavity through the jugular foramen. Here the fibres of the cranial root, which are derived from the nucleus ambiguus, join the vagus and are distributed with it. The fibres of the spinal root pass to the sternomastoid and trapezius muscles, which function to move the head and shoulders.

XII: HYPOGLOSSAL NERVE

The hypoglossal nerve is purely motor in function. It innervates both the extrinsic and intrinsic muscles of the tongue and, thus, serves to both move and change the shape of the tongue. The axons originate in the hypoglossal nucleus, which lies immediately beneath the floor of the fourth ventricle, near the midline (Fig. 7.16). Axons course ventrally through the medulla and

Cranial nerves

Cranial nerve	Component fibres	Structures innervated	Functions
I Olfactory	Sensory	Olfactory epithelium via olfactory bulb	Olfaction
II Optic	Sensory	Retina	Vision
III Oculomotor	Motor	Superior, inferior and medial rectus, inferior oblique, levator palpebrae muscles	Movement of the eyeball
	Parasympathetic	Pupillary constrictor and ciliary muscle of the eyeball, via ciliary ganglion	Pupillary constriction and accommodation
IV Trochlear	Motor	Superior oblique muscle	Movement of the eyeball
V Trigeminal	Sensory	Face, scalp, cornea, nasal and oral cavities, cranial dura mater	General sensation
	Motor	Muscles of mastication Tensor tympani muscle	Opening and closing the mouth Tension on tympanic membrane
VI Abducens	Motor	Lateral rectus muscle	Movement of the eyeball
VII Facial	Sensory	Anterior two-thirds of tongue	Taste
	Motor	Muscles of facial expression Stapedius muscle	Facial movement Tension on bones of middle ear
	Parasympathetic	Salivary and lacrimal glands via submandibular and pterygopalatine ganglia	Salivation and lacrimation
VIII Vestibulocochlear	Sensory	Vestibular apparatus	Vestibular sensation (position and movement of head)
		Cochlea	Hearing
IX Glossopharyngeal	Sensory	Pharynx, posterior third of tongue	General sensation and taste
		Eustachian tube, middle ear	General sensation
		Carotid body and carotid sinus	Chemo- and baroreception
	Motor	Stylopharyngeus muscle	Swallowing
	Parasympathetic	Parotid salivary gland via otic ganglion	Salivation
X Vagus	Sensory	Pharynx, larynx, oesophagus, external ear	General sensation
		Aortic bodies, aortic arch	Chemo- and baroreception
		Thoracic and abdominal viscera	Visceral sensation
	Motor	Soft palate, pharynx, larynx, upper oesophagus	Speech, swallowing
	Parasympathetic	Thoracic and abdominal viscera	Control of cardiovascular system, respiratory and gastro-intestinal tracts
XI Accessory	Motor	Sternomastoid and trapezius muscles	Movement of head and shoulder
XII Hypoglossal	Motor	Intrinsic and extrinsic muscles of the tongue	Movement of the tongue

Fig. 7.16 **Transverse section through the medulla**.
The diagram shows the origin and course of the fibres of the hypoglossal nerve.

emerge from its ventrolateral aspect as a linear series of rootlets located between the pyramid and the olive. The hypoglossal nucleus receives afferents from the nucleus solitarius and the trigeminal sensory nucleus; these are involved in the control of the reflex movements of chewing, sucking and swallowing. It also receives corticobulbar fibres from the contralateral motor cortex which subserve voluntary movements of the tongue, such as occur in speech.

Motor neurone disease and IX–XII nerve lesions

In motor neurone disease, a chronic degenerative disorder of the over-fifties, the corticobulbar tracts projecting to the nucleus ambiguus and hypoglossal nucleus degenerate leading to dysphonia (difficulty in phonation), dysphagia (difficulty in swallowing), dysarthria (difficulty in articulation), weakness and spasticity of the tongue (**pseudobulbar palsy**). There is also degeneration of the nucleus ambiguus and hypoglossal nuclei themselves leading to dysphonia, dysphagia, dysarthria and weakness, wasting and fasciculation of the tongue (**bulbar palsy**).

The ninth, tenth, eleventh and twelfth nerves can be damaged by compression in their peripheral course as they exit the cranium via the foramina of the skull base. Tumours in this area lead to dysphonia, unilateral weakness, wasting and fasciculation of the tongue and depression of the gag reflex, together with unilateral wasting of the sternomastoid and trapezius muscles.

Cerebellum

The cerebellum is the largest part of the hindbrain. It originates from the dorsal aspect of the brain stem and overlies the fourth ventricle. The cerebellum is connected to the brain stem by three stout pairs of fibre bundles, the **inferior, middle** and **superior cerebellar peduncles** (Fig. 8.1), which join the cerebellum to the medulla, pons and midbrain, respectively. The functions of the cerebellum are entirely motor and it operates at an unconscious level. It controls the maintenance of equilibrium (balance), influences posture and muscle tone and it coordinates movement.

EXTERNAL FEATURES OF THE CEREBELLUM

The cerebellum consists of two laterally located **hemispheres**, joined in the midline by the **vermis** (Figs 8.2–8.4). The superior surface of the cerebellum lies beneath the tentorium cerebelli and the superior vermis

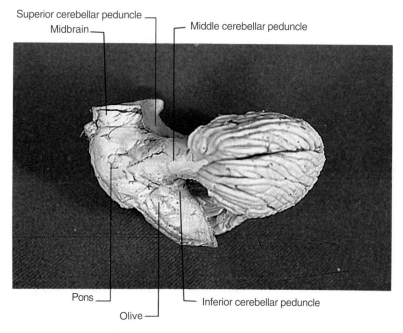

Fig. 8.1 **Lateral aspect of the brain stem and cerebellum, showing the cerebellar peduncles**.
Parts of the anterior, posterior and flocculonodular lobes have been removed to display the peduncles more clearly.

is raised, forming a midline ridge. Conversely, the inferior vermis lies in a deep groove between the hemispheres. The surface of the cerebellum is highly convoluted, the folds, or **folia**, being oriented approximately transversely. In between the folia lie fissures of varying depths. Some of these fissures are landmarks upon the basis of which the cerebellum is divided anatomically into three lobes (Figs 8.2–8.5): on the su-

perior surface, the deep **primary fissure** separates the relatively small **anterior lobe** from the much larger **posterior lobe**. On the underside, the conspicuous **posterolateral fissure** demarcates the location of small regions of the hemisphere (the **flocculus**) and vermis (the **nodule**), which together form the flocculonodular lobe.

Fig. 8.2 **Superior surface of the cerebellum**.

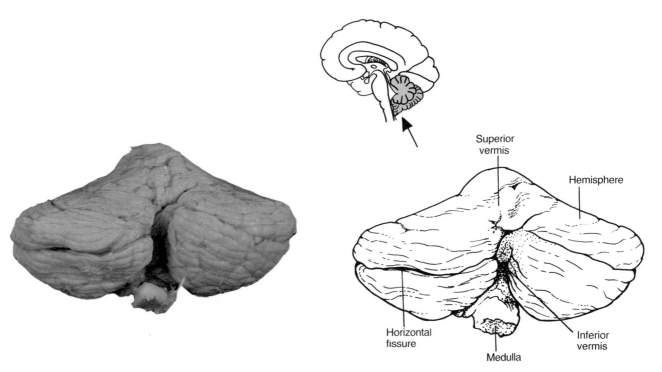

Fig. 8.3 **Posterior aspect of the cerebellum**.

Fig. 8.4 **Antero-inferior aspect of the cerebellum**.

Anterior lobe

Superior cerebellar
peduncle

Middle cerebellar
peduncle

Posterolateral
fissure

Inferior
cerebellar
peduncle

Posterior
lobe

Nodule   Flocculus

Flocculonodular
lobe

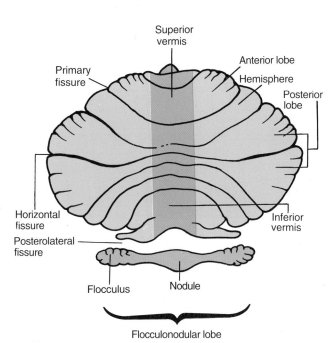

Superior
vermis

Primary
fissure

Anterior lobe

Hemisphere

Posterior
lobe

Horizontal
fissure

Posterolateral
fissure

Inferior
vermis

Flocculus   Nodule

Flocculonodular lobe

Fig. 8.5 **Schematic drawing of the cerebellum in which the peduncles have been cut and the surface flattened out**.
The relationships between the anatomical and functional divisions of the cerebellum are shown. (Green = archicerebellum; blue = paleocerebellum; pink = neocerebellum.)

External features of the cerebellum

- The cerebellum controls the maintenance of equilibrium, posture and muscle tone and it coordinates movement. It operates at an unconscious level.
- The cerebellum is connected to the medulla, pons and midbrain by the inferior, middle and superior cerebellar peduncles, respectively.
- The cerebellum consists of a midline vermis and two laterally located hemispheres.
- Anatomically, it is divided into anterior, posterior and flocculonodular lobes.

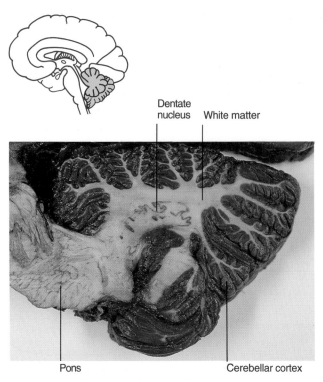

Dentate nucleus — White matter

Pons — Cerebellar cortex

Fig. 8.6 **Parasagittal section through the cerebellum**. Mulligan's stain.

INTERNAL STRUCTURE OF THE CEREBELLUM

The cerebellum basically consists of an outer layer of grey matter, the **cerebellar cortex**, and an inner core of white matter. The white matter is made up largely of afferent and efferent fibres which run to and from the cortex and towards which it extends irregular, branchlike projections (Fig. 8.6). Buried deep within the white matter are four pairs of **cerebellar nuclei** (Figs 8.6 and 8.9), which have important connections with the cerebellar cortex and with certain nuclei of the brain stem and thalamus.

CEREBELLAR CORTEX

The cerebellar cortex is highly convoluted, forming numerous transversely oriented folia. Within the cortex lie the cell bodies, dendrites and synaptic connections of the vast majority of cerebellar neurones. The cellular organisation of the cortex is the same in all regions (Fig. 8.7). It is divided histologically into three layers:

White matter — Molecular layer

Granular layer — **A** (× 25)

Purkinje cell layer — Molecular layer

Granular layer — **B** (× 60)

Molecular layer

Purkinje cell

Granular layer

C (× 160)

Fig. 8.7 **Transverse sections of cerebellar folia**. Illustration shows the layers of the cerebellar cortex.

- the outer, fibre rich, **molecular layer**
- the intermediate, **Purkinje cell layer**
- the inner, **granular layer**, which is dominated by the **granule cell**.

Afferent projections to the cerebellum arise principally from the spinal cord (spinocerebellar), inferior olivary nucleus (olivocerebellar), vestibular nuclei (vestibulocerebellar) and pons (pontocerebellar). Afferent fibres mostly terminate in the cortex where they are excitatory to cerebellar cortical neurones. Fibres enter the cerebellum through one or other of the cerebellar peduncles and proceed to the cortex as either **mossy fibres** or **climbing fibres** (Fig. 8.8). All afferents, other than those from the inferior olivary nucleus, end as mossy fibres. Mossy fibres branch to supply several folia and end in the granular layer, in synaptic contact with granule cells. The axons of granule cells pass towards the surface of the cortex and enter the molecular layer. Here they bifurcate to produce two **parallel fibres** which are oriented along the long axis of the folium.

The Purkinje cell layer consists of a unicellular layer of the somata of Purkinje neurones. The profuse dendritic arborisations of these cells (see Fig. 2.1B) extend towards the surface of the cortex, into the molecular layer (Fig. 8.8). The arborisations are flattened and oriented at right angles to the long axis of the folium. They are, therefore, traversed by numerous parallel fibres, from which they receive excitatory synaptic input. Inhibitory modulation of intracortical circuitry is provided by numerous other neurones known as Golgi, basket and stellate cells. The axons of Purkinje cells are the only axons to leave the cerebellar cortex. The great majority of these fibres do not leave the cerebellum entirely, but end in the deep cerebellar nuclei. The other type of afferent fibre entering the cerebellar cortex, the climbing fibre, originates from the inferior olivary nucleus of the medulla. These fibres provide relatively discrete excitatory input to Purkinje cells. At the same time, axon collaterals of climbing fibres excite the neurones of the deep cerebellar nuclei. Purkinje cells utilise GABA as their neurotransmitter, which means that the output of almost the whole of the cerebellar cortex is mediated through the inhibition of cells in the cerebellar nuclei.

CEREBELLAR NUCLEI

Deep within the cerebellar white matter, above the roof of the fourth ventricle, lie four pairs of nuclei. From medial to lateral, they are known as:

- **fastigial nucleus**
- **globose nucleus**
- **emboliform nucleus**
- **dentate nucleus** (Figs 8.6 and 8.9).

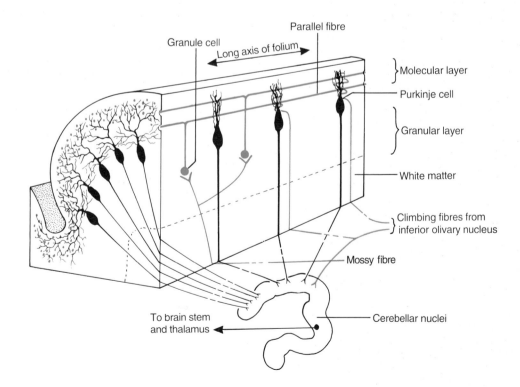

Fig. 8.8 **The cerebellar cortex.**
Diagram shows afferent and efferent connections and their relationships to the principal cells of the cortex.

Fig. 8.9 **Transverse section through the cerebellum and brain stem at the level of the fourth ventricle, showing the cerebellar nuclei.**

The dentate nucleus is by far the largest and is the only one which can be discerned clearly with the naked eye (Fig. 8.6). It consists of a thin layer of nerve cells folded into a crinkled bag and, thus, it appears somewhat similar to the inferior olivary nucleus of the medulla, from which it receives afferent fibres. The cerebellar nuclei also receive extracerebellar afferents from the vestibular nuclei, reticular nuclei, pontine nuclei and spinocerebellar tracts, predominantly by means of collaterals of mossy fibres destined for the cerebellar cortex. From within the cerebellum, the nuclei receive dense innervation from the Purkinje cells of the cerebellar cortex itself. The cerebellar nuclei constitute the primary source of efferent fibres from the cerebellum to other parts of the brain. The principal destinations of efferent fibres are the reticular and vestibular nuclei of the medulla and pons, the red nucleus of the midbrain and the ventral lateral nucleus of the thalamus.

Internal structure of the cerebellum

- Internally, the cerebellum consists of a surface layer of cortex, highly convoluted to form folia, beneath which lies white matter.
- Within the white matter lie cerebellar nuclei (fastigial, globose, emboliform and dentate).
- The nuclei are the origin of cerebellar efferent fibres.

Fig. 8.10 **Connections of the archicerebellum.**
Contralateral projections of the fastigial nucleus are not shown.

FUNCTIONAL ANATOMY OF THE CEREBELLUM

The cerebellum is often regarded as consisting of three functional subdivisions, based upon phylogenetic, anatomical and functional considerations (Fig. 8.5):

- The **archicerebellum**, or oldest portion in phylogenetic terms, is equated with the **flocculonodular lobe** and the associated **fastigial** nuclei.
- The **paleocerebellum** approximates to the midline **vermis** and surrounding **paravermis**, together with the **globose** and **emboliform** nuclei.
- The **neocerebellum** comprises the remainder (and vast majority) of the **cerebellar hemisphere** and the **dentate nuclei**.

ARCHICEREBELLUM

The archicerebellum is primarily concerned with the maintenance of balance (equilibrium). It has extensive connections with the vestibular and reticular nuclei of the brain stem, through the inferior cerebellar peduncles (Fig. 8.10). Vestibular information is carried from the vestibular nuclei to the cortex of the ipsilateral flocculonodular lobe. Cortical efferent (Purkinje cell) fibres project to the fastigial nucleus which, in turn, projects back to the vestibular nuclei and to the reticular formation. A significant proportion of fastigial efferents cross to the contralateral side of the brain stem. The influence of the archicerebellum upon the lower motor system is, therefore, bilateral and principally mediated by means of descending vestibulospinal and reticulospinal projections.

PALEOCEREBELLUM

The paleocerebellum influences muscle tone and posture. Afferents consist principally of dorsal and ventral spinocerebellar tract neurones which carry information from muscle, joint and cutaneous receptors and enter the cerebellum through the inferior and superior cerebellar peduncles, respectively (Fig. 8.11). Fibres terminate largely in the cortex of the ipsilateral vermis and paravermis. Cerebellar cortical efferents from these areas pass to the globose and emboliform nuclei, and also to the fastigial nucleus. The globose and emboliform nuclei project via the superior cerebellar peduncle to the contralateral red nucleus of the midbrain where they influence the activity of cells giving rise to the descending rubrospinal tract.

NEOCEREBELLUM

The neocerebellum is concerned with muscular coordination including the trajectory, speed and force of movements. The principal afferent pathway consists of pontocerebellar fibres (Fig. 8.12). These originate in the pontine nuclei of the basal portion of the pons and cross to the opposite side, entering the cerebellum through its middle peduncle. Pontocerebellar neurones are influenced by widespread regions of the cerebral

---

Lesions of the cerebellum

A midline lesion of the cerebellum (such as a tumour) leads to loss of postural control, so that it is impossible to stand or sit without toppling over, despite preserved coordination of the limbs.

Because of the pattern of ipsilateral and decussated pathways which enter and leave the cerebellum, unilateral lesions of the cerebellar hemisphere cause symptoms on the same side of the body. This is in contrast to cerebral lesions (e.g. in the cerebral cortex, internal capsule or basal ganglia) which give rise to contralateral symptoms.

A unilateral cerebellar hemispheric lesion causes ipsilateral incoordination of the arm (**intention tremor**) and of the leg, causing an unsteady gait, in the absence of weakness or sensory loss.

Bilateral dysfunction of the cerebellum, caused by alcoholic intoxication, hypothyroidism, inherited cerebellar degeneration/ataxia, multiple sclerosis or non-metastatic disease causes slowness and slurring of speech (**dysarthria**), incoordination of both arms and a staggering, wide-based, unsteady gait (**cerebellar ataxia**).

Cerebellar lesions also impair coordination of eye movements and the eyes exhibit a to-and-fro motion (**nystagmus**), greatest in amplitude when gaze is directed to the same side as the lesion. Nystagmus is a very common feature of multiple sclerosis. The combination of nystagmus with dysarthria and intention tremor consitutes '**Charcot's triad**', which is highly diagnostic of the disease.

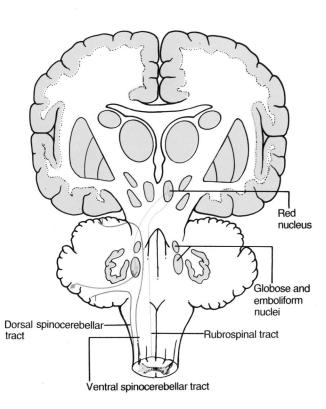

Fig. 8.11 **Connections of the paleocerebellum.**

Fig. 8.12 **Connections of the neocerebellum.**

cortex involved in the planning and execution of movement. Pontocerebellar fibres terminate predominantly in the lateral parts of the cerebellar hemisphere. Output from the neocerebellar cortex is directed to the dentate nucleus. The dentate nucleus in turn projects to the contralateral red nucleus and ventral lateral (VL) nucleus of the thalamus. The dentate is the largest of the cerebellar nuclei and its efferents form a major part of the superior cerebellar peduncle. The fibres decussate in the caudal midbrain just before reaching the red nucleus. Some relay in the red nucleus with rubro-thalamic cells but most bypass the red nucleus and pass directly to the VL thalamus. The ventral lateral nucleus of the thalamus projects to the cerebral cortex, particularly the motor cortex of the frontal lobe. The neocerebellum thus exerts its coordinating role in movement primarily through an action on cerebral cortical areas giving rise to descending corticospinal and corticobulbar pathways.

Functional anatomy of the cerebellum

- The archicerebellum corresponds to the flocculonodular lobe and fastigial nucleus. Its principal connections are with the vestibular and reticular nuclei of the brain stem and it is concerned with the maintenance of equilibrium.
- The paleocerebellum corresponds to the vermis and paravermal area, together with the globose and emboliform nuclei. It receives fibres from the spinocerebellar tracts and projects to the red nucleus of the midbrain.
- The neocerebellum corresponds to the majority of the cerebellar hemisphere and the dentate nucleus. It receives afferents from the pons and projects to the ventral lateral nucleus of the thalamus.
- Cerebellar lesions cause incoordination of the upper limbs (intention tremor), lower limbs (cerebellar ataxia), speech (dysarthria) and eyes (nystagmus).

Thalamus

Rostral to the midbrain lies the forebrain (prosencephalon, cerebrum; see Fig. 1.5). The forebrain consists of the bilaterally paired diencephalon and cerebral hemisphere on each side and is by far the largest derivative of the three basic embryological divisions of the brain. The diencephalon is continuous with the rostral part of the midbrain and lies in between the brain stem and cerebral hemisphere. The diencephalon comprises, from dorsal to ventral: the epithalamus, thalamus, subthalamus and hypothalamus, of which the thalamus is the largest. The thalamus consists of numerous nuclei, most of which have extensive reciprocal connections with the cerebral cortex. Of particular note are:

- nuclei which transmit general and special sensory information to corresponding regions of the sensory cortices
- nuclei which receive impulses from the cerebellum and basal ganglia and interface with motor regions of the frontal lobe
- nuclei which have connections with associative and limbic areas of the cortex.

The diencephalon is almost entirely surrounded by the cerebral hemisphere and, thus, little of its structure can be seen externally, apart from the ventral portion of the hypothalamus which can be seen on the base of the brain (Fig. 9.1). Immediately caudal to the optic chiasma is a small midline elevation, the **tuber cinereum**. From its apex, in life, extends the **infundibulum** or pituitary stalk which attaches to the pituitary gland. Caudal to the tuber cinereum, a pair of rounded eminences, the **mammillary bodies**, are located on

Optic chiasma

Optic tract

Optic nerve

Infundibulum

Tuber cinereum

Oculomotor nerve

Crus cerebri

Mammillary body

Fig. 9.1 **Ventral aspect of the diencephalon**.

either side of the midline. These contain the mammillary nuclei of the **hypothalamus**. The hypothalamus lies below the thalamus, extending medial and ventral to the subthalamus. It has important connections with the limbic system, a controlling influence upon the activity of the autonomic nervous system and a central role in neuroendocrine function, partly through its relationship with the pituitary gland. The hypothalamus receives further discussion in Chapter 13.

The other parts of the diencephalon can be seen in sagittal and coronal sections of the brain (Figs 9.2 and 9.3). The diencephalon forms the lateral wall of the third ventricle. The dorsal part of the ventricular wall is formed by the thalamus and the ventral part by the hypothalamus. The **epithalamus** is a relatively small part of the diencephalon and is located in its most caudal and dorsal region, immediately rostral to the superior colliculus of the midbrain. It consists principally of the **pineal gland** and the **habenular nuclei**. The pineal gland is an endocrine organ. It synthesises the hormone melatonin. The pineal gland has been implicated in control of the sleep/waking cycle and in regulation of the onset of puberty. The habenular nuclei have connections with the limbic system (Ch. 13).

The **subthalamus** lies beneath the thalamus and dorsolateral to the hypothalamus, with its ventrolateral aspect against the internal capsule. It contains two notable cell groups, the subthalamic nucleus and the zona incerta. The subthalamic nucleus is located in the ventrolateral part of the subthalamus, immediately medial to the internal capsule. It has the shape of a biconvex lens in coronal section. The subthalamic nucleus has prominent connections with the globus pallidus and the substantia nigra and is important in the control of movement. It is discussed in more detail in Chapter 11. The zona incerta is a rostral extension of the brain stem reticular formation. Several important fibre systems traverse the subthalamus en route to the thalamus. These include ascending sensory projections (medial lemniscus, spinothalamic tracts, trigeminothalamic tracts), cerebellothalamic fibres from the dentate nucleus and pallidothalamic fibres from the medial segment of the globus pallidus. The latter envelop the zona incerta as the lenticular fasciculus and thalamic fasciculus.

TOPOGRAPHICAL ANATOMY OF THE THALAMUS

EXTERNAL FEATURES

The thalamus has been likened in size and shape to a small hen's egg. Together with the hypothalamus it forms the lateral wall of the third ventricle, the transition between the two being marked by a faint groove,

Fig. 9.2 **Median sagittal section of the brain showing the relationships of the diencephalon**.

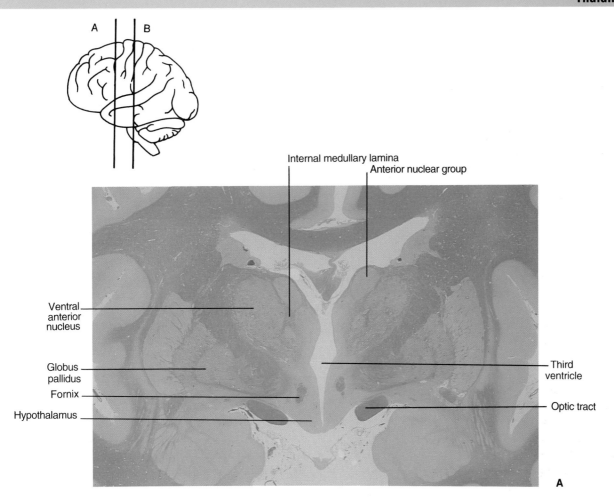

Internal medullary lamina
Anterior nuclear group

Ventral anterior nucleus

Globus pallidus

Fornix

Hypothalamus

Third ventricle

Optic tract

A

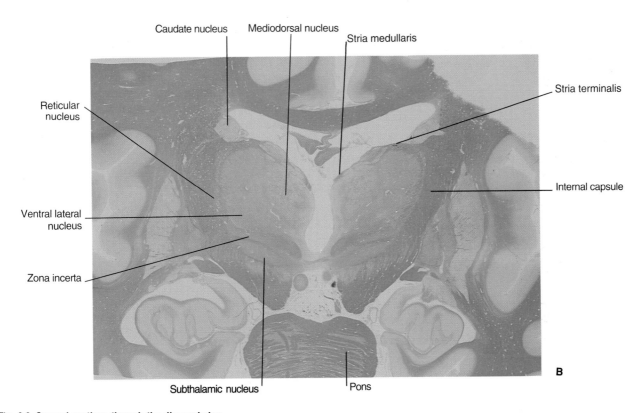

Caudate nucleus   Mediodorsal nucleus   Stria medullaris

Reticular nucleus

Stria terminalis

Internal capsule

Ventral lateral nucleus

Zona incerta

Subthalamic nucleus   Pons

B

Fig. 9.3 **Coronal sections through the diencephalon**.
Luxol fast blue stain for myelin.

the hypothalamic sulcus. In most individuals the two thalami are joined, across the thin slit of the ventricle, by the **interthalamic adhesion** or **massa intermedia**. A fascicle of nerve fibres, the **stria medullaris**, which has limbic connections, courses along the dorsomedial margin of the thalamus (Fig. 9.2). Along this line, the ependymal lining of the third ventricle spans the narrow lumen to form the ventricular roof.

The anterior pole of the thalamus extends as far as the interventricular foramen, through which the third and lateral ventricles are in continuity. Lateral to the thalamus lies the posterior limb of the internal capsule and anterolateral lies the head of the caudate nucleus (Fig. 9.4). The dorsal aspect of the thalamus thus forms part of the floor of the body of the lateral ventricle. Another fascicle of nerve fibres with limbic connections, the **stria terminalis**, marks the boundary between thalamus and caudate (Fig. 9.4). Ventral to the thalamus lie the subthalamus and hypothalamus; caudal to it lies the midbrain.

INTERNAL ORGANISATION

Within the thalamus is located a thin layer of nerve fibres composed of some of the afferent and efferent connections of thalamic nuclei. This is called the **internal medullary lamina** (Figs 9.3, 9.5 and 9.6). The lamina is roughly Y-shaped, when viewed from above, and provides the basis for dividing the majority of the thalamus into three nuclear masses: **anterior, medial** and **lateral**. Each of these cellular complexes is further subdivided into a number of individually named nuclei. Embedded within the internal medullary lamina are several cell groups, known collectively as the **intralaminar nuclei** (Fig. 9.6). Lateral to the main mass of thalamic nuclei lies another sheet of nerve fibres, the **lateral medullary lamina**, which consists of thalamocortical and corticothalamic fibres. Between this and the internal capsule is located a thin stratum of neurones which constitute the **reticular nucleus** of the thalamus (Fig. 9.3).

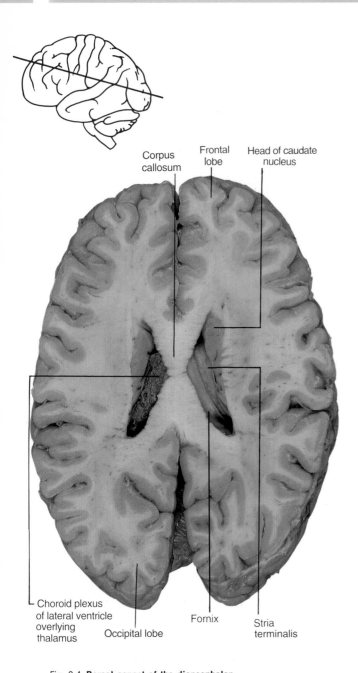

Fig. 9.4 **Dorsal aspect of the diencephalon**.
The choroid plexus has been removed on the right side.

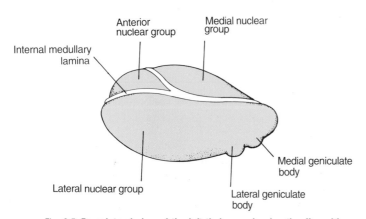

Fig. 9.5 **Dorsolateral view of the left thalamus showing the disposition of the internal medullary lamina and the principal nuclear divisions**.

Anatomy of the thalamus

- The thalamus is the largest component of the diencephalon, which is situated between the brain stem and the cerebral hemisphere.
- Almost all thalamic nuclei have rich reciprocal connections with the cerebral cortex.
- The thalamus is divided into three principal nuclear masses (anterior, medial and lateral) by the internal medullary lamina.
- Embedded within the internal medullary lamina lie intralaminar nuclei.
- On the lateral aspect of the thalamus lies the thin reticular nucleus.

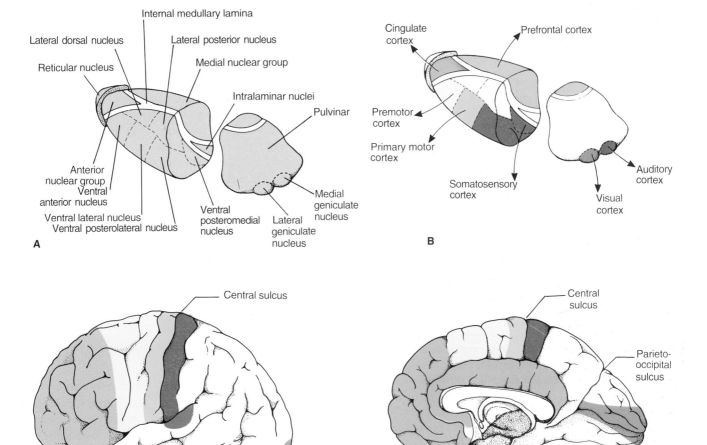

Fig.9.6 **Organisation of thalamic nuclei and their principal relationships with the cerebral cortex.**
The thalamus is viewed from its posterolateral aspect. The posterior part has been sectioned from the rest to reveal the internal structure. In (**A**) the principal thalamic nuclei are identified and in (**B**) their efferent connections are indicated. Colours represent the interrelationships between thalamic nuclei and cerebral cortical regions on the lateral (**C**) and medial (**D**) aspects of the cerebral hemisphere.

FUNCTIONAL ORGANISATION OF THALAMIC NUCLEI

All the nuclei of the thalamus, with the exception of the reticular nucleus, project to the ipsilateral cerebral cortex and the whole of the cortex receives input from the thalamus. Similarly, all thalamic nuclei receive corticofugal fibres in a basically reciprocal fashion. In some cases, precise, point-to-point projections exist between individual thalamic nuclei and restricted cortical zones with well-defined sensory or motor functions. This typifies the relationship between the thalamic nuclei and cortical regions which subserve the general and special senses, and the motor regions which receive cerebellar and basal ganglia input.

Such thalamic nuclei are often referred to as the **'specific' nuclei**. The specific nuclei all lie within the ventral part (tier) of the lateral nuclear group. Other nuclei receive less functionally distinct afferent input, which does not include overtly sensory or motor pathways, and connect with wider areas of cortex, including associative and limbic domains. These are often referred to as the **'non-specific' nuclei**. Non-specific nuclei include the nuclei of the dorsal tier of the lateral nuclear complex as well as the whole of the anterior and medial complexes.

Thalamic lesions

Strokes and tumours destroying the thalamus lead to loss of sensation in the contralateral face and limbs, accompanied by a distressing discomfort in the paradoxically anaesthetic areas (**thalamic pain**). Thalamic lesions may mimic cortical focal defects because of the richness of thalamocortical connections.

LATERAL NUCLEAR GROUP

The lateral nuclear group contains all of the so-called 'specific' thalamic nuclei. These are located in the ventral part of the complex and include the ventral anterior, ventral lateral, ventral posterior, lateral geniculate and medial geniculate nuclei (Fig. 9.6).

Ventral posterior (VP) nucleus

The ventral posterior nucleus lies between the ventrolateral nucleus and the pulvinar. Within VP thalamus terminate all of the ascending pathways from the spinal cord and brain stem which carry general sensory information from the contralateral half of the body to a conscious level. These pathways include the spinothalamic tracts, medial lemniscus and trigemino-thalamic tracts. The termination of these fibres in the VP nucleus is highly organised somatotopically.

The large lateral portion of the nucleus which receives information from the trunk and limbs (via the spinothalamic tracts and medial lemniscus) is referred to as the ventral posterolateral (VPl) division of VP, whilst a smaller, medial, portion which receives information from the head (via the trigeminothalamic tract) is termed the ventral posteromedial nucleus (VPm). In addition, taste information from the nucleus solitarius of the medulla and vestibular information from the vestibular nuclei reach the VPm thalamus. The ventral posterior nucleus projects to the primary somatosensory cortex in the postcentral gyrus of the parietal lobe.

Lateral geniculate nucleus (LGN)

The geniculate nuclei are located near the posterior pole of the thalamus, ventral to the pulvinar. Here they form small eminences on the surface, known as the geniculate bodies. The lateral geniculate nucleus is a part of the visual system and receives further discussion in Chapter 12.

It is the site of termination of the optic tract which carries the axons of retinal ganglion cells. Due to hemidecussation of optic nerve fibres in the optic chiasma, each nucleus receives axons which have originated in the ipsilateral temporal hemiretina and the contralateral nasal hemiretina. Thus, each nucleus receives visual information relating to the contralateral half of the visual field. The lateral geniculate nucleus sends fibres, via the retrolenticular part of the internal capsule and the optic radiation, to the primary visual cortex of the occipital lobe.

Medial geniculate nucleus (MGN)

The medial geniculate nucleus is part of the auditory system, which is described in Chapter 7. It receives ascending fibres from the inferior colliculus of the midbrain, via the inferior brachium. The medial geniculate nucleus projects, via the retrolenticular part of the internal capsule and the auditory radiation, to the primary auditory cortex of the temporal lobe.

Ventral anterior (VA) nucleus

The ventral anterior nucleus occupies the rostral part of the lateral nuclear mass. It consists of two subdivisions: the larger, principal part (VApc) and the smaller, magnocellular part (VAmc). The principal subcortical afferents to this region are output fibres of the ipsilateral basal ganglia system, which originate from the medial segment of the globus pallidus and its homologue, the pars reticulata of the substantia nigra. Fibres from the globus pallidus terminate in VApc whilst those from the substantia nigra end in VAmc. The VA thalamus has reciprocal connections with motor regions of the frontal lobe, particularly the premotor and supplementary motor cortices. It is, therefore, an important part of the mechanism by which the basal ganglia exert their influence on normal movement and through which abnormalities of movement are mediated in basal ganglia disorders.

Ventral lateral (VL) nucleus

The ventral lateral nucleus lies immediately caudal to VA in the ventral tier of the lateral nuclear complex. It consists of three subdivisions: pars oralis (VLo), pars medialis (VLm) and pars caudalis (VLc). Subcortical afferents to VL originate mainly from the ipsilateral globus pallidus and substantia nigra, and from the contralateral dentate nucleus of the cerebellum. Pallidal and nigral afferents terminate in VLo and VLm whilst those from the cerebellum terminate in VLc. The ventral lateral nucleus, like VA, has reciprocal connections with motor areas of the frontal lobe and especially with the primary motor cortex of the precentral gyrus.

> ### Surgical treatment of disorders of the basal ganglia
>
> Neurosurgically placed lesions in the region of the ventral anterior and ventral lateral nuclei have been used to alleviate some of the motor symptoms associated with disorders of the basal ganglia (rigidity, tremor at rest, dyskinesias) and cerebellum (intention tremor). Such **thalamotomy** has been largely superseded by drug therapy in basal ganglia disease, but is still used to relieve cerebellar tremor, e.g. in multiple sclerosis.

Within the dorsal tier of the lateral nuclear complex lie a number of so-called 'non-specific' nuclei. The lateral dorsal nucleus is part of the limbic system. It receives afferents from the hippocampus and sends

> **Functional organisation of the lateral nuclear group**
>
> - 'Specific' thalamic nuclei have well-defined sensory or motor functions and highly organised connections with sensory and motor regions of the cerebral cortex.
> - 'Non-specific' nuclei connect with wider areas of cortex, including associative and limbic regions.
>
> 'Specific' nuclei all lie within the ventral tier of the lateral nuclear mass. They include:
> - Ventral posterior nucleus: receives general sensory afferents in the medial lemniscus, spinothalamic tract and trigeminothalamic tract; sends efferents to the primary somatosensory cortex of the parietal lobe.
> - Lateral geniculate nucleus: receives visual afferents in the optic tract; projects to the primary visual cortex of the occipital lobe.
> - Medial geniculate nucleus: receives auditory afferents from the inferior colliculus; sends efferents to the primary auditory cortex of the temporal lobe.
> - Ventral anterior and ventral lateral nuclei: receive afferents from the cerebellum and basal ganglia; send efferents to motor cortical areas of the frontal lobe.

efferents to the cingulate gyrus. The lateral posterior nucleus has connections with the sensory association cortex of the parietal lobe. The **pulvinar** is a large region at the most posterior part of the thalamus. It has extensive connections with association cortices of the parietal, temporal and occipital lobes.

ANTERIOR NUCLEAR GROUP

The most anterior portion of the thalamus, extending to its rostral pole, is the anterior nuclear complex. It consists of three subdivisions: the anteroventral, anteromedial and anterodorsal nuclei, the individual connections of which will not be discussed. The anterior nuclear group is part of the limbic system. It receives a large afferent projection from the mammillary body of the hypothalamus via the mammillothalamic tract. The anterior complex projects principally to the cingulate gyrus on the medial surface of the cerebral hemisphere. It is involved in the control of instinctive drives, the emotional aspects of behaviour and in memory.

MEDIAL NUCLEAR GROUP

This large region consists primarily of the mediodorsal nucleus (MD or dorsomedial nucleus) and some much smaller components, such as the nucleus reuniens. Subcortical afferents to the mediodorsal nucleus come from

the hypothalamus, amygdala and from other thalamic nuclei, including the intralaminar nuclei and nuclei of the lateral complex. Extensive reciprocal connections exist between the mediodorsal nucleus and the prefrontal cortex. It is concerned mainly with the control of mood and the emotions.

INTRALAMINAR NUCLEI

Several nuclei lie embedded within the internal medullary lamina of the thalamus. These include the centromedian and parafascicular nuclei, the centromedian being the largest intralaminar nucleus in man. The intralaminar nuclei receive ascending afferents from the brain stem reticular formation and also from the spinothalamic and trigeminothalamic systems. In turn, they project to widespread regions of the cerebral cortex and to the caudate nucleus and putamen of the basal ganglia. The intralaminar nuclei are part of the mechanism for activation of the cerebral cortical mantle. Their stimulation causes desynchronisation of the electroencephalogram (EEG) and disruption of alpha rhythm, which is associated with repose and sleep. Lesions of the intralaminar nuclei reduce the perception of pain and the level of consciousness.

RETICULAR NUCLEUS

The reticular nucleus is a thin layer of cells located on the lateral aspect of the thalamus, between the external medullary lamina and the internal capsule. This nucleus receives collaterals of both thalamocortical and corticothalamic fibres which pass between other thalamic nuclei and the cerebral cortex.

> **Functional organisation of anterior, medial, intralaminar and reticular nuclei**
>
> - The anterior nuclear group of the thalamus is part of the limbic system. This region receives fibres from the mammillary body of the hypothalamus and projects to the cingulate gyrus.
> - Within the medial nuclear group, the mediodorsal nucleus has extensive reciprocal connections with the cortex of the frontal lobe.
> - The intralaminar nuclei receive input from the reticular formation and ascending sensory systems. They project to the cerebral cortex and the striatum and are responsible for activation of the cerebral cortex.
> - The reticular nucleus receives collaterals of thalamocortical and corticothalamic fibres.

Cerebral hemisphere and cerebral cortex

The cerebral hemisphere is derived from the embryological telencephalon (p. 5). It is the largest part of the forebrain and it reaches the greatest degree of development in the human brain. Superficially, the cerebral hemisphere consists of a layer of grey matter, the cerebral cortex, which is highly convoluted to form a complex pattern of ridges (gyri) and furrows (sulci). This serves to maximise the surface area of the cerebral cortex, about 70% of which is hidden within the depths of sulci (Figs 10.1 and 10.2). Beneath the surface, axons

Fig. 10.1 **Lateral aspect of the cerebral hemisphere showing major gyri and sulci.**

Fig. 10.2 **Median sagittal section of the cerebral hemisphere showing major gyri and sulci.**
The brain stem and cerebellum have been removed to show the inferomedial aspect of the temporal lobe.

Corpus callosum

Head of caudate nucleus

Anterior horn of lateral ventricle

Fig. 10.3 **Coronal section of the brain.**

Head of caudate nucleus

Anterior limb of internal capsule

Fig. 10.4 **Coronal section.**

Corpus callosum

Anterior horn of lateral ventricle

Temporal lobe

Septum pellucidum

Fig. 10.5 **Coronal section.**

running to and from the cells of the cortex form an extensive mass of white matter (Figs 10.3–10.12). The vast majority of those nerve fibres which pass between the cerebral cortex and subcortical structures are condensed, deep within the hemisphere, into a broad sheet called the **internal capsule** (Figs 1.13 and 10.4–10.11). Between the internal capsule and the cortical surface, fibres radiate in and out to produce a fan-like arrangement, the **corona radiata**. Buried within the white matter lie a number of nuclear masses, most notably the caudate nucleus, putamen and globus pallidus, known collectively as the basal ganglia (Figs 10.3–10.15). Within the cerebral hemisphere lies the large C-shaped cavity of the lateral ventricle, which is

considered with the rest of the ventricular system in Chapter 15.

The two cerebral hemispheres are separated by a deep cleft, the **great longitudinal fissure**, which accommodates the meningeal **falx cerebri**. In the depths of the fissure, the hemispheres are united by the **corpus callosum**, an enormous sheet of commissural nerve fibres which run between corresponding areas of the two cortices (Figs 10.2–10.15, 10.22 and 10.23).

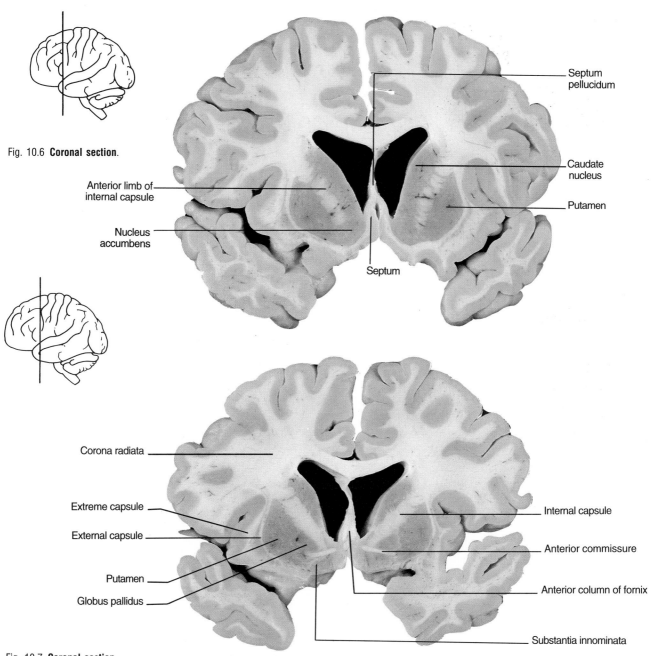

Fig. 10.6 **Coronal section**.

Septum pellucidum

Anterior limb of internal capsule

Caudate nucleus

Nucleus accumbens

Putamen

Septum

Corona radiata

Extreme capsule

External capsule

Internal capsule

Anterior commissure

Putamen

Anterior column of fornix

Globus pallidus

Substantia innominata

Fig. 10.7 **Coronal section**.

Fornix

Caudate nucleus

Lateral medullary lamina

Globus pallidus
  lateral segment

Lateral fissure

Claustrum

  medial segment

Hippocampus

Amygdala

Mammillary body

Fig. 10.8 Coronal section.

Insula

Internal capsule

Tail of caudate nucleus

Thalamus

Hippocampus

Third ventricle

Subthalamic nucleus

Substantia nigra

Fig. 10.9 Coronal section.

Great longitudinal fissure

Fornix

Thalamus

Inferior horn of lateral ventricle

Red nucleus

Crus cerebri

Substantia nigra

Fig. 10.10 Coronal section.

GYRI, SULCI AND LOBES OF THE CEREBRAL HEMISPHERE

Certain gyri and sulci on the surface of the hemisphere are consistently located in different individuals and form the basis of dividing the hemisphere into four lobes, namely the **frontal**, **parietal**, **temporal** and **occipital lobes**. Their principal topographical features are described below and their functional significance is considered in more detail on page 110. The most conspicuous and deepest cleft on the lateral surface of the hemisphere is the **lateral fissure** (Fig. 10.1). This separates the temporal lobe below, from the frontal and parietal lobes above. Within the depths of the lateral fissure lies a cortical area known as the **insula**

(Figs 10.6–10.14). Parts of the frontal, parietal and temporal lobes which overlie the insula are called the **opercula**. Also on the lateral surface of the hemisphere, a single, uninterrupted sulcus can usually be identified, running continuously between the great longitudinal fissure and the lateral fissure. This is the **central sulcus**, which marks the boundary between the frontal and parietal lobes (Figs 10.1 and 10.16). The central sulcus extends for a short distance onto the medial surface of the hemisphere, within the great longitudinal fissure (Figs 10.2 and 10.16).

The frontal lobe constitutes the entire region in front of the central sulcus. Immediately in front of the sulcus, and running parallel to it, lies the **precentral gyrus**, which is the primary motor region of the cerebral cortex (p. 110). In front of the precentral gyrus, the rest of

Lateral fissure

Tail of caudate nucleus

Temporal lobe

Lateral geniculate nucleus

Habenula

Posterior commissure

Pons

Fig. 10.11 **Coronal section**.

Pulvinar

Hippocampus

Brachium conjunctivum

Fornix

Pineal gland

Pedunculopontine nucleus

Cerebral aqueduct

Fig. 10.12 **Coronal section**.

the frontal lobe consists of a more variable pattern of convolutions, of which the **superior**, **middle** and **inferior frontal gyri** can usually be identified (Fig. 10.1).

Behind the central sulcus, and above the lateral fissure, lies the parietal lobe. Its most anterior part is the **postcentral gyrus**, which is the site of the primary somatosensory cortex (p. 111). Behind the postcentral gyrus, on the lateral surface of the hemisphere, the **intraparietal sulcus** divides the rest of the parietal

lobe into superior and inferior parietal lobules (Figs 10.1 and 10.16).

The boundary between the parietal lobe and the posteriorly located occipital lobe is not coincident with a single sulcus on the lateral surface of the hemisphere but, on the medial surface, it is clearly marked by the deep **parieto-occipital sulcus** (Figs 10.2 and 10.16). The occipital lobe does not bear any important landmarks on its lateral surface but, on the medial surface,

Fig. 10.13 **Horizontal (axial) magnetic resonance image of the living brain**. (Courtesy of Dr. A. Jackson, Department of Diagnostic Radiology, University of Manchester.)

Rostrum of corpus callosum

Anterior limb of internal capsule

Head of caudate nucleus

Insula

Extreme capsule

External capsule

Putamen

Claustrum

Posterior limb of internal capsule

Globus pallidus

Retrolenticular part of internal capsule

Thalamus

Tail of caudate nucleus

Splenium of corpus callosum

Fig. 10.14 **Horizontal section of the brain**.

Fig. 10.15 **Coronal magnetic resonance image of the living brain**.
(Courtesy of Dr. A. Jackson, Department of Diagnostic Radiology, University of Manchester.)

Fig. 10.16 **(A)** Lateral aspect of the cerebral hemisphere showing major functional areas.
(B) Median sagittal section of the cerebral hemisphere showing major functional areas.

the prominent **calcarine sulcus** indicates the location of the primary visual cortex (Figs 10.2 and 10.16).

The temporal lobe lies beneath the lateral fissure, merging posteriorly with the parietal and occipital lobes. On its lateral surface the temporal lobe is divided into three principal gyri which run parallel to the lateral fissure: the superior, middle and inferior temporal gyri (Fig. 10.1). The superior temporal gyrus includes the primary auditory cortex. Most of this functional region is situated on the superior bank of the gyrus, within the lateral fissure, where the **transverse temporal gyri**, or **Heschl's convolutions**, provide a more precise localisation (Fig. 10.21).

On the medial surface of the hemisphere, certain portions of the frontal, parietal and temporal lobes also constitute components of the limbic system. Curving around the corpus callosum, and running parallel to it, lies the **cingulate gyrus** (Figs 10.2 and 10.16), separated from the rest of the hemisphere by the **cingulate sulcus**. The cingulate gyrus passes posteriorly and inferiorly round the posterior portion, or splenium, of the corpus callosum, to become continuous with the **parahippocampal gyrus** of the temporal lobe. Deep to the parahippocampal gyrus, within the temporal lobe, lies the **hippocampus** (Figs 10.8–10.12). This structure is formed by an in-curling of the inferomedial part of the temporal lobe. The cingulate gyrus, parahippocampal gyrus and hippocampus are sometimes referred to as the **limbic lobe** of the cerebral hemisphere.

CEREBRAL CORTEX

HISTOLOGICAL STRUCTURE

The cerebral cortex is a layer, several millimetres in thickness, consisting of nerve cell bodies, dendritic arborisations and synaptic interconnections which forms the outer surface of the cerebral hemisphere. In the early part of this century, Brodmann produced a numbered cytoarchitectural map of the cerebral cortex based upon histological characteristics. Although largely superseded by functional considerations, in some instances there is good correspondence between **Brodmann's areas** and functionally defined regions of the cortex. In such cases, Brodmann's numbers are retained in common use for descriptive purposes.

Long ago in evolutionary history, the cerebral cortex originally arose in relation to olfactory function. Phylogenetically old parts of the cortex (referred to as **archicortex** and **paleocortex**), such as the hippocampus and other parts of the temporal lobe, retain throughout evolution an association with the olfactory system and have a primitive, three-layered cytoarchitecture. These regions have important functions in the emotional aspects of behaviour and in memory. Together with other parts of the cortex and certain subcortical nuclei they constitute the limbic system (Ch. 13). The majority of the cerebral cortex is a more recent acquisition in phylogenetic terms and is referred

---

Gyri, sulci and lobes of the cerebral hemisphere

- The cerebral hemisphere consists of:
  - the superficial cerebral cortex, convoluted to form gyri and sulci
  - underlying white matter, consisting of cortical afferent and efferent fibres
  - deep nuclear masses, the basal ganglia.
- The two cerebral hemispheres are separated by the great longitudinal fissure and joined by the corpus callosum.
- The hemisphere is divided into four lobes (frontal, parietal, temporal and occipital) on the basis of surface topography.
- Principal landmarks which indicate the divisions between lobes are: the lateral fissure, central sulcus and parieto-occipital sulcus.

Fig. 10.17 **The histological structure of the cerebral cortex.** (From Mitchell and Patterson, *Basic Anatomy*, 1954, courtesy of Churchill Livingstone.)

Layer

I

II

III

IV

V

VI

White matter

to as the **neocortex**. Although its detailed cytological structure varies from region to region it is generally recognised as consisting of six layers (Fig. 10.17).

- **Layer I** the most superficial layer, contains few nerve cell bodies but many dendritic and axonal processes in synaptic interaction.
- **Layer II** contains many small neurones which establish intracortical connections.
- **Layer III** contains medium-sized neurones giving rise to association and commissural fibres.
- **Layer IV** is the site of termination of afferent fibres from the specific thalamic nuclei.
- **Layer V** is the origin of projection fibres to extracortical targets, such as basal ganglia, thalamus, brain stem and spinal cord. In the primary motor cortex of the frontal lobe this layer contains the giant Betz cells which project fibres into the pyramidal tract.
- **Layer VI** also contains association and projection neurones.

FUNCTIONAL ORGANISATION

The cerebral cortex is necessary for conscious awareness and thought, memory and intellect. It is the region to which all sensory modalities ultimately ascend (mostly via the thalamus) and where they are consciously perceived and interpreted in the light of previous experience. The cerebral cortex is the highest level at which the motor system is represented. It is here that actions are conceived and initiated.

- The posterior cerebrum receives sensory information from the outside world in the primary sensory areas of the parietal lobe (somatosensory), occipital lobe (vision) and temporal lobe (hearing).
- In adjacent cortical zones the information is elaborated to permit identification of objects by touch, sight and hearing in a modality specific act of perception. Areas of cortex at the junction of the three cerebral lobes, known as association cortex, are critical

---

Focal cerebral lesions

Focal cerebral lesions, e.g. a stroke or tumour, produce three kinds of symptoms:

- **Partial epileptic seizures**. The repetitive discharges of groups of neurones in the cerebral cortex produce paroxysmal attacks lasting for brief periods and reflecting the functional properties of the neurones concerned. The patient experiences sudden attacks of abnormal movements or sensations (**simple partial seizures**) or brief alterations in perception, mood and behaviour (**complex partial seizures**). Partial seizures may trigger **generalized (tonic–clonic) seizures**.
- **Sensory/motor deficits**. There is a loss of sensation or movement, detectable on clinical neurological examination.

- **Psychological deficits**. There are breakdowns in psychological processes such as language, perception and memory, demonstrable on psychological evaluation.

If the focal lesion is space-occupying, the syndrome of **raised intracranial pressure** results (see p. 32).

A **unilateral cerebral hemisphere lesion** causes mental impairment (e.g. aphasia), a contralateral spastic hemiparesis, hyperreflexia and an extensor plantar response (upper motor neurone lesion) and contralateral hemisensory loss (Fig. 10.18; see also Fig. 1.26). A vascular insult to the internal capsule, such as an infarction or haemorrhage, leads to the rapid development of this syndrome, known as a **stroke**.

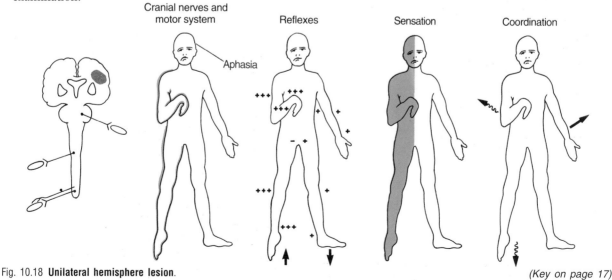

Fig. 10.18 **Unilateral hemisphere lesion.**
(Key on page 17)

for the multimodal and spatial recognition of the environment.

- The medial portions of the cerebral hemisphere (limbic system) enable the storage and retrieval of information processed in the posterior hemispheres.
- The anterior cerebrum (frontal lobes) is concerned with the organisation of movement (primary motor area, premotor and supplementary motor areas) and the strategic guidance of complex motor behaviour over time (prefrontal area).
- In the majority of individuals, areas of association cortex in frontal, parietal and temporal lobes of the left hemisphere are responsible for the comprehension and expression of language. The left hemisphere is, therefore, said to be dominant for language.

Frontal lobe

The frontal lobe lies anterior to the central sulcus. Immediately anterior to the central sulcus, and running parallel to it, is the precentral gyrus. Functionally, this is known as the **primary motor cortex** (Figs 10.1, 10.2 and 10.16). It corresponds to Brodmann's area 4. Within the cortex of the precentral gyrus the contralateral half of the body is represented in a somatotopic fashion, often pictorially depicted as a 'motor homunculus' (Fig. 10.19). The representation of the body is inverted, with the head area located in the most inferior part of the precentral gyrus, just above the lateral fissure. Progressing superiorly, areas of cortex are encountered in which are successively represented the digits, hand, arm, shoulder and trunk. The lower limb is represented on the medial surface of the hemisphere. The area of cortex devoted to a particular body part is proportionate not to its size but to the degree of precision with which movements can be executed. Thus, the larynx, tongue, face and digits of the hand are represented by relatively large regions.

Stimulation of the primary motor cortex elicits contraction of discrete muscle groups on the opposite side of the body. The function of this region is the control of voluntary, skilled movements, sometimes referred to as fractionated movements; 30% of corticospinal (pyramidal tract) and corticobulbar fibres arise from neurones of the primary motor cortex, about 3% originating from giant pyramidal (Betz) cells. The principal subcortical afferents to the primary motor cortex originate from the ventral lateral nucleus of the thalamus (Fig. 9.6, p. 97) which in turn receives input mainly from the dentate nucleus of the cerebellum and from the globus pallidus of the basal ganglia.

The region immediately anterior to the primary motor cortex is known as the **premotor cortex** (Brodmann's area 6) (Fig. 10.16). On the lateral surface of the hemisphere, this includes the posterior portions of the superior, middle and inferior frontal gyri. On the medial surface of the hemisphere, the premotor cortex includes a region referred to as the **supple-mentary motor cortex**. Here, like the primary motor cortex, there is somatotopic representation of the body although, unlike the primary motor cortex, representation appears to be bilateral in both hemispheres.

Stimulation of premotor cortical areas induces movements which are less focused than those elicited from primary motor cortex and which involve groups of functionally related muscles. Movements evoked from the supplementary motor cortex tend to be postural in nature, involving axial and proximal musculature. Premotor cortical areas are thought to function in the programming of, and preparation for, movement and in the control of posture. The premotor cortex exerts its actions partly via the primary motor cortex, with which it is connected by short association fibres, and partly via corticospinal and corticobulbar fibres. About 30% of the latter originate in the premotor cortex although, unlike the primary motor cortex, giant Betz cells are absent from premotor areas. The principal subcortical input to premotor cortical regions, including the supplementary motor cortex, is the ventral anterior nucleus of the thalamus. This, in turn, receives fibres from the globus pallidus and substantia nigra.

Immediately in front of the premotor cortex, on the lateral surface of the hemisphere, are located two other important regions. In the middle frontal gyrus, lies the **frontal eye field** (Brodmann's area 8). This region controls voluntary conjugate deviation of the eyes, as occur when scanning the visual field. Unilateral damage to this area causes conjugate deviation of the eyes towards the side of the lesion. In the inferior frontal gyrus of the dominant hemisphere (usually the left), lies the motor speech area, also known as **Broca's area** (Brodmann's areas 44 and 45). Broca's area has important interconnections with parts of the ipsilateral temporal, parietal and occipital lobes which are involved in language function.

The extensive regions of the cortex of the frontal

Left frontal lobe lesions

Lesions of the left frontal lobe lead to:

- Partial seizures: paroxysmal jerking movements of the contralateral limbs are termed 'simple motor' or **'Jacksonian' seizures**.
- Sensory/motor deficit: weakness of the face and upper motor neurone signs in the limbs on the opposite side to the lesion (**contralateral hemiplegia**).
- Psychological deficit: speech is produced with great effort and poor articulation, in brief utterances with word errors (paraphasia). Repetition of words is impaired but powers of comprehension are relatively preserved. This is known as **Broca's aphasia**. There is also impairment of reading and writing (**alexia** and **agraphia**).

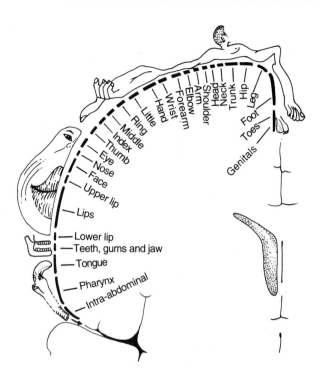

Fig. 10.19 **Motor homunculus illustrating somatotopic organisation of the primary motor cortex.**
(Modified from Penfield and Rasmussen, *The Cerebral Cortex of Man: A Clinical Study of Localization of Function*, 1950, courtesy of MacMillan.)

Fig. 10.20 **Sensory homunculus illustrating somatotopic organisation of the primary somatosensory cortex.**
(Modified from Penfield and Rasmussen, *The Cerebral Cortex of Man: A Clinical Study of Localization of Function*, 1950, courtesy of MacMillan.)

lobe which lie anterior to premotor areas are referred to as **prefrontal cortex**. The prefrontal cortex has rich connections with parietal, temporal and occipital cortex through long association fibres running in the subcortical white matter. Subcortical afferents arise mainly in the mediodorsal and anterior nuclei of the thalamus. The prefrontal cortex has cognitive functions of a high order. These include intellectual, judgmental and predictive faculties and the planning of behaviour.

Bilateral cortical disorders

Alzheimer's disease, a common degenerative disorder of the elderly, leads to atrophy of the temporal and parietal lobes and the limbic system. It causes disorientation in space, loss of language (**aphasia**) and memory (**amnesia**).

In **general paralysis of the insane** (GPI) due to neuro-syphilitic infection, both frontal lobes are destroyed and there is total alteration of personality with loss of judgement, planning and insight and bizarre and uncharacteristic behaviour. The less common degenerative disorder of fronto-temporal **lobar atrophy**, including **Pick's disease**, causes personal and social misconduct similar to GPI.

Parietal lobe

The parietal lobe lies behind the frontal lobe and is bounded posteriorly and inferiorly by the occipital and temporal lobes, respectively. The most anterior part of the parietal lobe is the postcentral gyrus, running parallel to the central sulcus (Figs 10.1, 10.2 and 10.16). Functionally, this region is the **primary somatosensory cortex** (Brodmann's areas 1, 2 and 3). It is here that thalamocortical neurones terminate which constitute the third and final neurone in the chain from peripheral receptors for general sensation to a conscious level. The thalamic origin of these neurones is the ventral posterior nucleus, which in turn receives fibres of the medial lemniscus (fine touch and proprioception), spinal lemniscus (coarse touch and pressure), spinothalamic tracts (pain and temperature) and trigeminothalamic tracts (general sensation from the head). Within the somatosensory cortex the contralateral half of the body is represented in an inverted, somatotopic pattern which resembles that in the primary motor cortex of the frontal lobe (Fig. 10.20).

Once again, the area of cortex devoted to a particular body part is disproportionate to its size but, rather, reflects the richness of sensory innervation. Thus, the pharynx, tongue, face, lips and the palmar surface of the hands and digits are particularly well represented. Adjacent to the mouth area is a region where taste is perceived.

The surface of the parietal lobe posterior to the primary somatosensory cortex constitutes the parietal **association cortex**. The superior parietal lobule is responsible for the interpretation of general sensory information and for conscious awareness of the contralateral half of the body. Lesions here impair the interpretation and understanding of sensory input and may cause neglect of the opposite side of the body. The inferior parietal lobule interfaces between somato-sensory cortex and the visual and auditory association cortices of the occipital and temporal lobes, respectively, and in the dominant hemisphere contributes to language functions.

Left parietal lobe lesions

- Partial seizures: paroxysmal attacks of abnormal sensations, spreading down the contralateral side of the body (sensory seizures).
- Sensory/motor deficit: a contralateral hemisensory loss and inferior visual field loss.
- Psychological deficit: an inability to name objects (**anomia**) and a loss of literacy, with inability to read (alexia), to write (agraphia) and to calculate (**acalculia**).

Right parietal lobe lesions

- Partial seizures: paroxysmal attacks of sensory disturbance affect the contralateral side of the body (simple sensory seizures).
- Sensory/motor deficit: contralateral hemisensory loss and an inferior visual field loss.
- Psychological deficit: an inability to copy and construct designs because of spatial disorientation (**constructional apraxia**).

Temporal lobe

The lateral surface of the temporal lobe is divided into superior, middle and inferior temporal gyri, which run parallel to the lateral fissure. Within the superior temporal gyrus is located the **primary auditory cortex** (Brodmann's areas 41 and 42). More exactly, the majority of this functional zone lies in the superior bank of the gyrus, normally hidden within the lateral fissure. Its precise location is marked by the small transverse temporal gyri, or Heschl's convolutions (Fig. 10.21).

The primary auditory cortex is responsible for the conscious perception of sound and within it there is so-called tonotopical representation of the cochlear duct. It receives input from the medial geniculate nucleus of the thalamus. The ascending acoustic projection undergoes partial decussation in the brain stem on its way to the medial geniculate nucleus (p. 81). At the cortical level, therefore, the organs of hearing are bilaterally represented so that unilateral lesions of the primary auditory cortex cause partial deafness in both ears. Auditory information is further processed and interpreted in the **auditory association cortex**, which lies immediately posterior to the primary auditory cortex. In the dominant hemisphere this region is also known as **Wernicke's area**. It is crucial for understanding of

Frontal pole

Occipital pole

Temporal pole

Insula

Transverse temporal gyri

Fig. 10.21. **Lateral aspect of the cerebral hemisphere**.
The frontal and parietal operculae have been removed to show the location of the transverse temporal gyri (Heschl's convolutions) and the insula.

Left temporal lobe lesions

• Partial seizures: paroxysmal attacks of un-responsiveness (**absences**), purposeless behaviour (**automatism**), olfactory and complex visual and auditory hallucinations and disturbances of mood and memory (**déja vu**). These attacks are referred to as complex partial seizures.
• Sensory/motor deficit: a contralateral superior visual field loss.
• Psychological deficit: speech is fluent and rapid but contains word errors (paraphasia) and is incomprehensible. There is profound word-finding difficulty, impaired repetition of words, and profound loss of comprehension. This is known as **Wernicke's aphasia**.

Occipital lobe lesions

• Partial seizures: paroxysmal visual hallucinations of a simple, unformed nature, such as lights and colours (simple partial seizures).
• Sensory\motor deficit: a contralateral visual field loss (**contralateral homonymous hemianopia**).

Bilateral occipital lobe lesions lead to **cortical blindness** of which the patient is unaware (**Anton's syndrome**). Bilateral occipito–parietal lesions can spare elementary vision but prevent the recognition and depiction of objects (**apperceptive visual agnosia**).

---

the spoken word and it has important connections with other language areas of the brain.

The location of the cortical representation of the vestibular system is uncertain. There is evidence that it lies in the superior temporal gyrus, anterior to the primary auditory cortex, or in the inferior parietal lobule.

The inferomedial part of the temporal lobe is curled inwards to form the **hippocampus**. This structure lies in the floor of the inferior horn of the lateral ventricle, deep to the parahippocampal gyrus (Figs 10.8–10.12, 10.16 and Ch. 13). As part of the limbic system, the principal functions of the hippocampus are in relation to memory and the emotional aspects of behaviour. Close to the anterior end of the hippocampus and the temporal pole lies a mass of subcortical grey matter, the **amygdala**, which is also part of the limbic system. The amygdala and adjacent parts of the inferomedial temporal cortex receive fibres from the olfactory tract and are responsible for the conscious appreciation of the sense of smell. These connections receive further consideration in Chapter 13.

Occipital lobe

The occipital lobe lies behind the parietal and temporal lobes. On the medial surface of the hemisphere, the boundary with the parietal lobe is marked by the deep parieto-occipital sulcus. Also on the medial surface, the calcarine sulcus marks the location of the **primary visual cortex** (Brodmann's area 17) (Fig. 10.16), which is responsible for visual perception. It occupies the gyri immediately above and below the calcarine sulcus, much of it being hidden in the depths of the sulcus. This region receives fibres from the lateral geniculate nucleus of the thalamus, by way of the optic radiation of the internal capsule. Each lateral half of the visual field is represented in the primary visual cortex of the contralateral hemisphere. The upper half of the visual field is represented below the calcarine sulcus,

and the lower half above the sulcus. The rest of the occipital lobe constitutes the **visual association cortex**. This region is concerned with the interpretation of visual images. Lesions of the primary visual cortex cause blindness in the corresponding part of the visual field, whilst damage to the visual association cortex causes deficits in visual interpretation and recognition.

Language areas of the cerebral hemisphere

Certain higher cognitive functions are dealt with primarily, or even exclusively, by one of the cerebral hemispheres, which is then referred to as dominant for that function. In the great majority of people the left hemisphere is dominant for language and mathematical ability. The right hemisphere excels at spatial perception and musical proficiency. Cerebral dominance becomes established during the first few years after birth. During this formative period, both hemispheres exhibit linguistic ability and if one hemisphere sustains damage it may be compensated for, by the plasticity of the developing brain, so that the child learns to speak normally. Later in life this flexibility becomes greatly diminished and damage to the dominant hemisphere often causes loss of speech, in addition to the other deficits produced by hemispheric lesions.

The language areas of the brain are organised around the lateral fissure of the cerebral hemisphere. In the frontal lobe, Broca's area occupies the posterior part of the inferior frontal gyrus, adjacent to the motor cortical area for the head and neck. This region is concerned with expressive aspects of language. In the temporal lobe, the auditory association cortex, or Wernicke's area, is responsible for comprehension of the spoken word.

Nearby regions of the temporal lobe and parietal lobe, most notably the angular gyrus and supramarginal gyrus of the inferior parietal lobule, provide a functional interface between auditory and visual association areas important in naming, reading, writing and calculation.

The cerebral cortex

- The precentral gyrus is the primary motor region of the cerebral cortex located within the frontal lobe, immediately in front of the central sulcus. Anterior to this lie the premotor and supplementary motor cortices and, in the left hemisphere, Broca's (motor speech) area. The prefrontal cortex is concerned with complex cognitive functions.
- The postcentral gyrus is the primary somatosensory region of the cerebral cortex and lies within the parietal lobe, immediately posterior to the central sulcus. It receives afferents from the ventral posterior nucleus of the thalamus which is the site of termination of the spinothalamic tracts, trigeminothalamic tract and the medial lemniscus. Behind this region lies the sensory association cortex which is responsible for the interpretation of general sensory information.
- The temporal lobe lies beneath the lateral fissure. On the superior surface of the superior temporal gyrus, the transverse temporal gyri (Heschl's convolutions) mark the location of the primary auditory cortex which receives input from the medial geniculate nucleus of the thalamus. Adjacent lies the auditory association cortex which is responsible for the interpretation of auditory information and which, in the left hemisphere, constitutes Wernicke's area.
- The occipital lobe makes up the posterior part of the hemisphere. On the medial surface, the calcarine sulcus indicates the location of the primary visual cortex which receives afferents from the lateral geniculate nucleus of the thalamus. The rest of the occipital lobe is the visual association cortex which is responsible for the interpretation of visual information.

WHITE MATTER OF THE CEREBRAL HEMISPHERE

Beneath the cortical surface lies an enormous mass of nerve fibres all of which have their origin or termination, or sometimes both, within the cortex. The fibres are classified, depending upon their origin and destination into:

- **Association fibres** which interconnect cortical sites lying within one cerebral hemisphere.
- **Commissural fibres** which run from one cerebral hemisphere to the other, connecting functionally related structures.
- **Projection fibres** which pass between the cerebral cortex and subcortical structures such as the thalamus, striatum, brain stem and spinal cord.

Association fibres

Some association fibres (Figs 10.22 and 10.23) are short and link nearby areas of cortex by arching beneath adjacent cerebral sulci (U fibres). Other association fibres are longer and travel through the white matter to link distant areas of cerebral cortex. The primary sensory areas in the parietal, temporal and occipital lobes are linked by long association fibres to the association areas of the cerebral cortex. These in turn are connected to each other.

The large **superior longitudinal fasciculus** interconnects the frontal and occipital lobes. A subsidiary of this bundle, known as the **arcuate fasciculus**, links gyri in the frontal and temporal lobes which are important for language function.

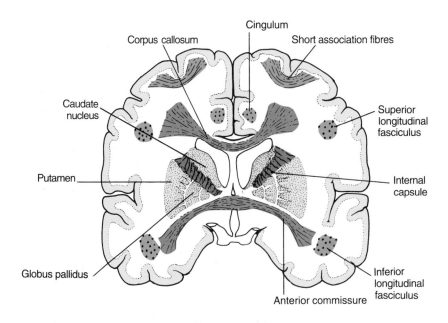

Fig. 10.22 **Coronal section of the cerebral hemisphere.**
The diagram shows the location of the principal association, commissural and projection fibres.

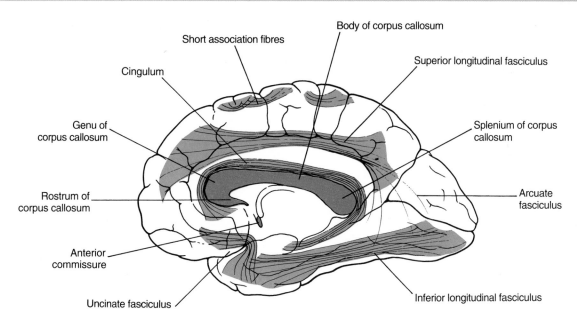

Fig. 10.23 **Principal association and commissural fibres of the cerebral hemisphere projected onto the medial surface.**

The **inferior longitudinal fasciculus** runs from the occipital to the temporal poles and contributes to the function of visual recognition.

Associative agnosia

Cerebral damage such as that caused by carbon monoxide poisoning can destroy the inferior longitudinal fasciculus bilaterally. In such cases the individual has intact elementary vision but cannot identify the nature of objects (**object agnosia**) or individual faces (**prosopagnosia**) but can depict and match them.

The **uncinate fasciculus** connects the anterior and inferior parts of the frontal lobe with the temporal gyri which are important structures in the regulation of behaviour. The **cingulum** lies within the cingulate gyrus and courses around the corpus callosum, connecting the frontal and parietal lobes with the parahippocampal and adjacent temporal gyri.

Commissural fibres

The major interhemispheric commissural fibres are the corpus callosum, the anterior commissure and the hippocampal commissure, or commissure of the fornix (Figs 10.22–10.24).

The **corpus callosum** spans the two cerebral hemispheres and connects corresponding regions of neocortex for all but the temporal fields (these have their own connection, the anterior commissure). The major parts of the corpus callosum, from rostral to caudal, are the rostrum, genu, body and splenium. The corpus callosum is shorter rostrocaudally than is the hemisphere so that callosal fibres linking the frontal or occipital poles curve forwards or backwards as the anterior and posterior forceps, respectively. The **splenium** interconnects the occipital cortices and, therefore, contributes to visual functions.

Damage to the corpus callosum

Patients with chronic epilepsy have undergone section of the corpus callosum to relieve their seizures. Such individuals betray few difficulties under normal circumstances. However, when these **'split-brain' patients** undergo psychological testing the two halves of the brain appear to behave relatively autonomously. For example, visual information directed to the right non-dominant hemisphere alone does not evoke a verbal response, so that individuals cannot name objects or read words presented solely to the left visual field.

Destruction of the splenium of the corpus callosum by stroke or tumour leads to the posterior disconnection syndrome of **alexia without agraphia**. Such individuals speak and write without difficulty but cannot understand written material (alexia). Disconnection of visual processing in the right hemisphere from the verbal processing of the dominant left hemisphere is thought to explain the syndrome.

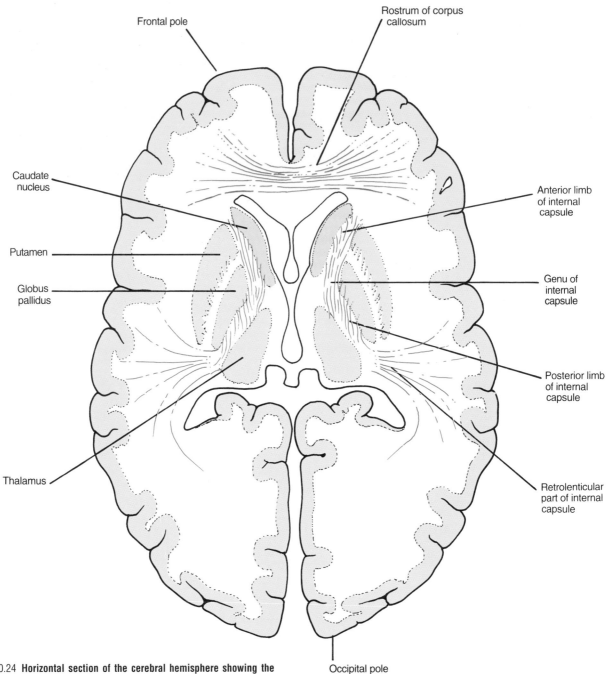

Fig. 10.24 **Horizontal section of the cerebral hemisphere showing the parts of the internal capsule**.

The **anterior commissure** runs transversely in front of the anterior column of the fornix and interconnects the inferior and middle temporal gyri and the olfactory regions on the two sides.

The **hippocampal commissure** consists of transverse fibres linking the posterior columns of the fornix on each side.

Projection fibres

Projection fibres (Fig. 10.22) consist of afferent fibres conveying impulses to the cortex and efferent fibres conducting impulses away from it. The fibres projecting to and from the cerebral cortex are distributed radially as the corona radiata and then converge downwards towards the brain stem. The fibres become concentrated in a narrow area, called the **internal capsule**, between the thalamus and caudate nucleus medially, and the lentiform nucleus laterally. The internal capsule is angulated to form an anterior limb, genu, posterior limb and retrolenticular part (Fig. 10.24).

The **anterior limb** contains connections between the mediodorsal nucleus of the thalamus and the prefrontal cortex, and also frontopontine fibres which project to the pontine nuclei in the basal portion of the pons.

The **posterior limb** contains corticobulbar and corticospinal motor fibres. Also within the posterior limb are thalamocortical projections passing from the ventral posterior nucleus to the primary somatosensory cortex, and from the ventral anterior and ventral lateral nuclei to motor regions of the frontal lobe.

Behind the posterior limb is a region referred to as the **retrolenticular** part of the internal capsule. This consists of fibres arising from the medial and lateral geniculate nuclei of the thalamus which pass to the auditory and visual cortices as the auditory and visual radiations, respectively. Visual thalamocortical fibres (also known as geniculocalcarine fibres) pass round the lateral ventricle and follow one of two courses to the visual cortex. Those which represent the lower half of the visual field project to the upper part of the visual cortex (above the calcarine sulcus). They may be interrupted in their course by lesions of the parietal lobe. Fibres which represent the upper half of the visual field loop forwards over the inferior horn of the lateral ventricle (Meyer's loop) and may be damaged by lesions of the temporal lobe.

White matter of the cerebral hemisphere

- Nerve fibres within the subcortical white matter are classified on the basis of their origin and termination.
- Association fibres link cortical regions within a single hemisphere.
- Important systems of association fibres are: the superior longitudinal fasciculus, arcuate fasciculus, inferior longitudinal fasciculus and uncinate fasciculus.
- Commissural fibres pass between corresponding regions of the two hemispheres. The principal commissural system is the corpus callosum.
- Projection fibres run between the cerebral cortex and various subcortical structures. They pass through the corona radiata and the internal capsule.
- Particularly important fibres in this category are corticospinal, corticobulbar and thalamocortical projections.

Corpus striatum

Within the cerebral hemisphere lie a number of nuclear masses, collectively referred to as the **basal ganglia** (Figs 11.1, 10.3–10.9 and 10.14). The major components are the **caudate nucleus**, **putamen**, **globus pallidus** and **amygdala**. The amygdala, which is located within the temporal lobe, is part of the limbic system and is considered in Chapter 13.

The caudate nucleus, putamen and globus pallidus are anatomically and functionally closely related to each other and are principally involved in the control of posture and movement. They are sometimes referred to anatomically as the **corpus striatum** but, clinically, abnormalities of movement resulting from their dysfunction are commonly called basal ganglia disorders. The corpus striatum has important connections with other regions of the brain, particularly with the thalamus and subthalamic nucleus of the diencephalon and the substantia nigra of the midbrain.

Fig. 11.1 **Horizontal section of the brain illustrating the corpus striatum**.
Mulligan's stain has been used to increase the contrast between cell-rich areas (blue) and white matter.

Gross anatomically, the putamen and globus pallidus are sometimes together called the **lentiform** (or lenticular) **nucleus**. This is because they lie close together forming an apparently single structure. The name means 'lentil-shaped' but a closer analogy would be a Brazil nut or the segment of an orange. The lentiform nucleus is three-sided, having a convex lateral surface and two other surfaces which converge to a medial apex which lies against the genu of the corpus callosum. The term lentiform or lenticular is, however, rather archaic and of limited usefulness, although it is retained in certain anatomical names (such as the retrolenticular part of the internal capsule).

On phylogenetic, connectional and functional grounds the putamen is more closely allied to the caudate nucleus than to the globus pallidus. The globus pallidus is, in phylogenetic terms, the oldest part of the corpus striatum and is sometimes referred to as the **paleostriatum**. The abbreviation **pallidum** is more commonly used, particularly in composite terms for afferent and efferent connections, such as subthalamopallidal or pallidothalamic.

The caudate nucleus and putamen constitute the phylogenetically more recent **neostriatum** and are best regarded as a single entity. The two parts are almost (but not entirely) separated by the internal capsule but their gross anatomical separation is not as significant as their neuronal and functional similarities. They are commonly referred to simply as the **striatum**.

These rather confusing relationships are summarised below:

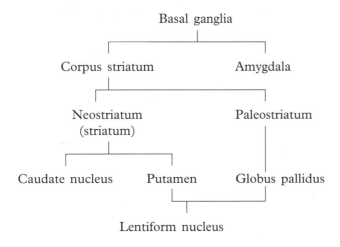

TOPOGRAPHICAL ANATOMY OF THE CORPUS STRIATUM

STRIATUM

The striatum (neostriatum) consists of the caudate nucleus and the putamen. Their combined three-dimensional shape is reminiscent of a tadpole, when viewed laterally (Fig. 11.2).

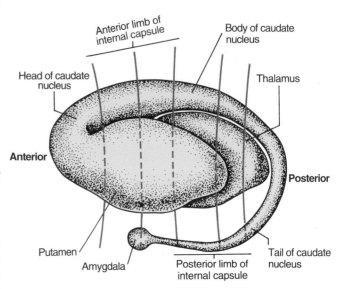

Fig. 11.2 **Lateral aspect of the left caudate nucleus, putamen, amygdala and thalamus.**
(The globus pallidus is obscured by the putamen.) The course of the internal capsule is shown in red. The putamen and the head of the caudate nucleus are separated by the anterior limb of the internal capsule, except at their most rostral extent where the two are in continuity. The posterior limb of the internal capsule separates the globus pallidus and putamen from the thalamus. (Modified with permission from Carpenter MB, Sutin J 1983 *Human Neuroanatomy*, 8th edn. Williams and Wilkins, Baltimore).

Putamen

The putamen lies lateral to the internal capsule and globus pallidus (Fig. 11.1 and Figs 10.7, 10.8 and 10.14). It is separated from the globus pallidus by a thin lamina of nerve fibres, the lateral medullary lamina. Lateral to the putamen lies more white matter, sandwiched within which lies a thin sheet of grey matter, known as the claustrum. This separates the white matter into two layers, the external capsule and the extreme capsule (Fig. 11.1). Lateral to the extreme capsule lies the cortex of the insula, deep within the lateral fissure of the hemisphere.

Caudate nucleus

The caudate nucleus consists of a large head and a tapering, curved tail. The head of the caudate is almost completely separated from the putamen by the internal capsule. At its rostral extremity, however, it is continuous with the putamen through and beneath the anterior limb of the capsule (Fig. 11.2 and Figs 10.4–10.6). At this level, the most ventral portion of the striatum is known as the **nucleus accumbens**, which has connections with the limbic system. The head of the caudate nucleus forms a prominent bulge in the lateral wall of the anterior horn of the lateral ventricle (Fig. 11.1 and Figs 10.3–10.7). The tail of the caudate passes posteriorly, gradually tapering as it does so and, following the curvature of the ventricle, descends into the temporal lobe where it lies in the roof of the inferior horn (Fig. 11.2 and Figs 10.9–10.12).

GLOBUS PALLIDUS

The globus pallidus lies medial to the putamen, separated from it by the lateral medullary lamina. Its medial apex nestles into the lateral concavity of the internal capsule (Fig. 11.1). The globus pallidus consists of two segments, lateral and medial, which are divided by a thin sheet of fibres, the medial medullary lamina (Fig. 11.1). The smaller medial segment shares many cytological and connectional similarities with the pars reticulata of the substantia nigra of the midbrain. Although the two are separated by the internal capsule, they are best regarded as a single entity, in the functional sense.

SUBSTANTIA INNOMINATA

The term substantia innominata refers to the basal part of the rostral forebrain which lies beneath the corpus striatum (Figs 10.7 and 11.5). This complex region contains several groups of neurones, one of them being the **nucleus basalis** (of Meynert), which project widely to the cerebral cortex and utilise acetylcholine as their neurotransmitter. These neurones undergo degeneration in Alzheimer's disease.

FUNCTIONAL ANATOMY OF THE CORPUS STRIATUM

CONNECTIONS OF THE STRIATUM

The caudate nucleus and putamen, together commonly referred to as the striatum, are best considered as a single entity, since they share common neuronal organisation, neurotransmitter systems and connections (Fig. 11.3). They are often regarded as the 'input' portions of the corpus striatum, since the majority of afferents from other parts of the brain end here, rather than in the globus pallidus.

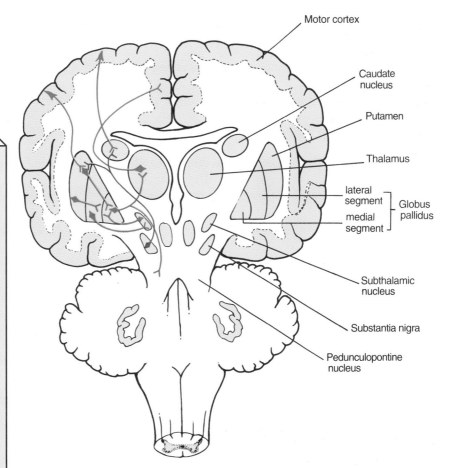

Topographical anatomy of the corpus striatum

- The corpus striatum includes the caudate nucleus, putamen and globus pallidus.
- These structures are primarily concerned with the control of posture and movement.
- Topographically the putamen and globus pallidus constitute the lentiform nucleus.
- Functionally the caudate nucleus and putamen form a single entity, the neostriatum (striatum), whilst the globus pallidus forms the paleostriatum.
- The caudate nucleus lies in the wall of the lateral ventricle.
- The largest part, or head, of the caudate lies medial to the internal capsule and forms a prominent bulge in the lateral wall of the anterior horn of the ventricle.
- The curved, tapering tail of the caudate follows the curvature of the lateral ventricle into the temporal lobe.
- The putamen and globus pallidus lie lateral to the internal capsule, deep to the cortex of the insula.

Fig. 11.3 **Schematic diagram illustrating the principal connections of the corpus striatum and related nuclei.**
Afferents to the striatum from the intralaminar thalamic nuclei and raphe nuclei have been omitted. For the sake of clarity, all efferents from the basal ganglia system are shown to originate from the medial segment of the globus pallidus, those from the pars reticulata of the substantia nigra being omitted. Similarly, efferents from the striatum are shown to originate only from the putamen and not from the caudate nucleus. Red: glutamatergic pathways; green: GABAergic pathways; purple: dopaminergic pathway.

Striatal afferents

Afferents to the striatum come from three principal sources: the cerebral cortex, the thalamus and the substantia nigra.

Corticostriatal fibres originate from widespread regions of the cerebral cortex, predominantly, but not exclusively, of the ipsilateral side. Fibres from the frontal and parietal lobes predominate. Motor regions of the frontal lobe project mainly to the putamen, where the body is represented in an inverted, somatotopic fashion. More anterior regions of the frontal lobe, and other association cortices, project mainly to the caudate nucleus. For these reasons, the putamen is considered to be the most obviously motor part of the striatum, the caudate nucleus having more associative functions. Corticostriatal fibres are excitatory to striatal neurones and use glutamic acid as their transmitter.

The **thalamostriatal projection** comes from the intralaminar nuclei (centromedian and parafascicular nuclei) of the ipsilateral thalamus.

The **nigrostriatal projection** originates from the **pars compacta** of the ipsilateral **substantia nigra** of the midbrain tegmentum. The transmitter used by this pathway is the monoamine dopamine, which has both excitatory and inhibitory effects upon striatal neurones. The neurones of the pars compacta contain the dark pigment neuromelanin which is produced as a by-product of dopamine synthesis (Fig. 11.4). The most rostral and ventral portion of the striatum, the nucleus accumbens, receives its dopaminergic input from the ventral tegmental area, which lies medial to the substantia nigra. This projection is known as the mesostriatal pathway. Other afferents to the striatum include a projection from the brain stem **raphe nuclei**, utilising 5-hydroxytryptamine (5-HT; serotonin) as their transmitter.

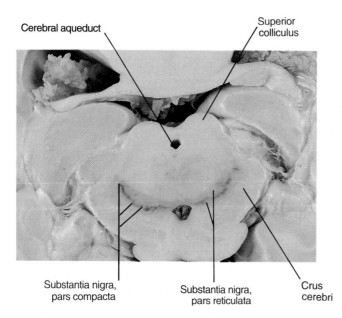

Fig. 11.4 **Transverse section through the midbrain showing the substantia nigra.**

Labels: Cerebral aqueduct; Superior colliculus; Substantia nigra, pars compacta; Substantia nigra, pars reticulata; Crus cerebri

Striatal efferents

The efferent projections of the striatum are directed principally to the two segments of the globus pallidus and to the pars reticulata of the substantia nigra (**striatopallidal** and **striatonigral fibres**, respectively). The cells of origin are so-called medium spiny neurones, which make up the majority of striatal nerve cells. Although there is some collateralisation, generally speaking, separate populations of neurones project to each of the three output targets (Fig. 11.3). These projections are inhibitory upon pallidal and nigral neurones and utilise GABA as their primary transmitter. In addition, a number of peptides are co-localised in these efferent neurones. The cells which project to the medial segment of the globus pallidus and the substantia nigra contain both **substance P** and **dynorphin**. The projection to the lateral segment of the globus pallidus contains **met-enkephalin**.

Connections of the striatum

- The caudate nucleus and putamen are the 'input' regions of the corpus striatum.
- They receive afferents from the cerebral cortex, intralaminar thalamic nuclei and the pars compacta of the substantia nigra.
- Efferent fibres are directed to the globus pallidus and the pars reticulata of the substantia nigra.

CONNECTIONS OF THE GLOBUS PALLIDUS

The two segments of the globus pallidus have similar afferent connections but substantially different efferent projections. The medial segment of the globus pallidus is very similar in structure and function to the pars reticulata of the substantia nigra, from which it is separated by the internal capsule. Together, the medial pallidum and pars reticulata of the substantia nigra are regarded as the 'output' portion of the basal ganglia, since they are the origin of the majority of basal ganglia efferent fibres that project to other levels of the neuraxis.

Pallidal afferents

Pallidal afferents arise principally from the striatum and from the subthalamic nucleus. Striatopallidal fibres are of two types, as previously noted, originating from different populations of striatal neurones. Both utilise GABA as their primary transmitter but, in addition each contains characteristic peptide co-transmitters. Fibres containing enkephalin project to the lateral pallidal segment, whilst those containing substance P and dynorphin project to the medial pallidum.

The **subthalamopallidal projection** originates in

the subthalamic nucleus of the caudal diencephalon (Fig. 11.5). This small structure is located beneath the thalamus, lying against the medial surface of the internal capsule. It has the appearance of a biconvex lens in coronal sections. Subthalamopallidal fibres pass laterally through the internal capsule, contributing to a fibre system known as the **subthalamic fasciculus,** and terminate in both segments of the globus pallidus, although termination is more dense in the medial segment.

The subthalamopallidal pathway is excitatory to pallidal neurones, using glutamic acid as its transmitter. The subthalamic nucleus also sends similar fibres to the pars reticulata of the substantia nigra, the other 'output' part of the basal ganglia system. The subthalamopallidal and subthalamonigral pathways are thought to have a pivotal role in the normal function of the basal ganglia and in the pathophysiology of basal ganglia disorders.

Fig. 11.5 **Coronal sections through the corpus striatum and diencephalon.** Luxol fast blue stain.

Pallidal efferents

The two pallidal segments have different efferent projections. The lateral segment projects principally to the subthalamic nucleus. Pallidosubthalamic fibres pass laterally through the internal capsule in the subthalamic fasciculus. This projection is inhibitory and uses GABA as its transmitter. The medial segment of the globus pallidus, together with the pars reticulata of the substantia nigra, projects primarily to the thalamus (ventral lateral (VL), ventral anterior (VA) and centromedian (CM) nuclei) with a smaller projection to the brain stem tegmentum. These output neurones are inhibitory and utilise GABA as their transmitter.

Pallidothalamic fibres take one of two routes (Fig. 11.6). Some pass round the anterior margin of the internal capsule as the **ansa lenticularis**, whilst others pass through the capsule as the **lenticular fasciculus**. The fibres continue to course medially and then loop dorsally and laterally as the **thalamic fasciculus**, to enter the thalamus from its ventral aspect. In following this trajectory, the fibres circumnavigate a cellular region of the subthalamus known as the **zona incerta**, which lies between the thalamus and the subthalamic nucleus.

Pallidothalamic fibres constitute the main outflow from the basal ganglia. Their thalamic target nuclei (VA and VL) in turn project excitatory fibres to the motor regions of the frontal lobe, principally the primary motor and supplementary motor cortices. A smaller contingent of medial pallidal efferent fibres passes caudally to terminate in the brain stem tegmentum in the **nucleus tegmenti pedunculopontinus** (pedunculopontine nucleus; PPN) which lies at the boundary between midbrain and pons, surrounding the superior cerebellar peduncle (Fig. 11.3 and Fig. 10.12). This region has been termed the **mesencephalic locomotor region** in lower mammals, since it is involved in the regulation of quadrupedal progression.

The pars reticulata of the substantia nigra is regarded as a homologue of the medial segment of the globus pallidus and to occupy a similar status with regard to the origin of basal ganglia output. Like the medial pallidum, the pars reticulata receives fibres from the striatum and the subthalamic nucleus. The projection from the striatum is somatotopically organised both in the pallidum and nigra such that the pallidal neurones are associated primarily with limb movements whereas nigral cells control the axial musculature, including the extraocular muscles. As already noted, efferents from the medial pallidum project to the VA/VL and CM thalamic nuclei and to the pedunculopontine nucleus. Efferents of the pars reticulata of the substantia nigra also pass to a subregion of the VL thalamus, superior colliculus and brain stem reticular formation (including the PPN).

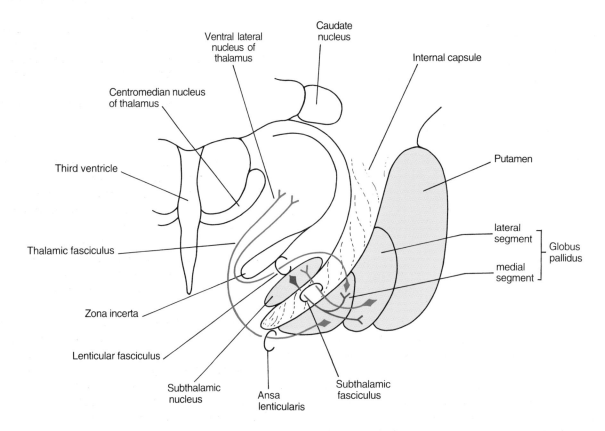

Fig. 11.6 **Schematic coronal section through the corpus striatum and diencephalon illustrating the efferent projections of the globus pallidus.** (Modified with permission from Carpenter MB, Sutin J 1983 *Human Neuroanatomy*, 8th edn. Williams and Wilkins, Baltimore.)

NORMAL FUNCTIONS OF THE BASAL GANGLIA

The basal ganglia are sometimes referred to as parts of the so-called 'extrapyramidal motor system'. This term was coined to distinguish the symptoms seen clinically in diseases of the basal ganglia, and related structures such as the substantia nigra and subthalamic nucleus, from those observed following stroke in the internal capsule, which were thought to be due to destruction of the pyramidal tract. As understanding of the functional anatomy of the motor system has increased, it has become apparent both that the pyramidal and extrapyramidal systems are intimately related rather than separate, and also that so-called pyramidal signs are not all attributable to dysfunction of the pyramidal tract itself. The term extrapyramidal is, therefore, somewhat outdated but is still in widespread use.

Current concepts of the role of the basal ganglia consider that their function is to facilitate behaviour and movements which are required and appropriate in any particular context and to inhibit unwanted or inappropriate behaviours\movements. How this might be achieved can be explained with reference to the internal connections of the basal ganglia (Fig. 11.3).

When a movement is initiated from the cerebral cortex, impulses discharge not only through corticospinal and corticobulbar pathways but also through the corticostriatal projection to the neostriatum. These glutamatergic fibres cause excitation of striatal neurones. The striatum has two routes by which it is able to control the activity of basal ganglia output neurones in the medial segment of the globus pallidus or the pars reticulata of the substantia nigra.

The first of these is the 'direct pathway', through which striatopallidal and striatonigral neurones will directly induce the inhibition of medial pallidal or pars reticulata neurones. This mechanism has been shown to operate in experimental electrophysiological studies

Basal ganglia syndromes

Unilateral basal ganglia lesions produce their effects on the opposite (contralateral) side of the body, as is the case with cerebral hemisphere lesions but distinct from cerebellar disorders. Basal ganglia dysfunction does not cause paralysis, sensory loss or ataxia, but leads to **abnormal motor control, alterations in muscular tone** and the emergence of abnormal, involuntary movements, or **dyskinesias**.

Abnormal motor control may consist of slowness of movement (**bradykinesia**) or poverty of movement (**hypokinesia, akinesia**). The initiation, sequencing and cessation of movement are disrupted. Normal posture cannot be maintained and 'associated' limb movements are lost, e.g. arm swinging when walking.

Tone may be increased throughout the range of passive movement (**rigidity**) and the hypertonia may be continuous (plastic) or discontinuous ('cogwheel'). Alternatively, **hypotonia** may occur.

Dyskinesias may be manifest in various ways and describe the abnormal movements, not the underlying disease. **Tremor** is a to-and-fro, sinusoidal movement which may be maximal at rest (resting tremor) or on action (action or postural tremor). **Chorea** is a sequence of rapid, asymmetrical, and fragmented (quasi-purposeful) movements usually affecting the distal limb musculature. **Dystonia** refers to sustained muscular contractions which give rise to abnormal postures or contortions. **Athetosis** consists of slow, sinuous, writhing movements. Sometimes movements share more than one characteristic, hence the term **choreo-athetosis**). **Myoclonus** describes sudden, shock-like movements, which are usually bilateral and especially affect the upper limbs. **Tics** are stereotyped movements, often highly characteristic of the individual, sometimes multiple and frequently influenced by emotional stress.

in primates where basal ganglia output neurones associated with a particular body part or muscle group show a pause in their action potential discharge during movement of that region (this has been shown for limb movements in the medial pallidum and eye movements in the substantia nigra, pars reticulata). Since medial pallidal and pars reticulata output neurones are themselves inhibitory, this leads to disinhibition of target neurones, including those of the motor thalamus. The resulting increase in the activity of thalamic neurones causes excitation of the cells of the cerebral cortex. The effect of activation of the direct pathway is, therefore, to support or facilitate ongoing movements.

The second route by which striatal neurones can influence the output of the basal ganglia is the so-called 'indirect pathway', via the subthalamic nucleus. Efferents from the striatum terminate in the lateral pallidal segment and their activation induces inhibition of lateral pallidal neurones. The principal efferent projection of the lateral pallidum is to the subthalamic nucleus which, thus, becomes disinhibited. The resultant increase in discharge of subthalamic neurones causes activation of medial pallidal and nigral neurones and, in turn, inhibition of thalamic and cortical cells. This has the effect of inhibiting unwanted movements.

PATHOPHYSIOLOGY OF BASAL GANGLIA DISORDERS

Studies on the post-mortem brains of patients with **Parkinson's disease** and experimental animal studies have provided insight into the pathophysiological mechanisms which underlie the appearance of parkinsonian symptoms (Fig. 11.7). Normally, dopamine apparently exerts an excitatory influence upon striatal neurones of the 'direct' projection to the medial pallidal segment and an inhibitory effect upon neurones of the 'indirect' pathway which projects to the lateral pallidal segment.

Loss of striatal dopamine, therefore, causes abnormal underactivity of the direct pathway and disinhibition of medial pallidal neurones. Simultaneously, overactivity of the indirect projection leads to inhibition of lateral pallidal neurones, disinhibition of the subthalamic nucleus, and thus excessive excitatory drive of medial pallidal cells. Changes in both the direct and indirect pathways, thus, compound to exacerbate the abnormal overactivity of medial pallidal output cells, inducing akinesia.

The archetypal basal ganglia disease in which dyskinesias occur is **Huntington's disease**. Within the striatum, there is particular attrition of the cells which project to the lateral segment of the globus pallidus (the 'indirect' projection), at least early on in the condition. This leads to disinhibition of lateral pallidal neurones and inhibition of the subthalamic nucleus (Fig. 11.7). Medial pallidal neurones thus become abnormally underactive and unwanted, involuntary movements ensue.

Fig. 11.7 **Schematic diagram illustrating how activities in basal ganglia and related nuclei become disordered in parkinsonism and chorea**.
Overactive pathways are emboldened; underactive pathways are interrupted. Labelling as for Figure 11.3.

Basal ganglia diseases

Parkinson's disease is a neurodegenerative disease, usually of the elderly, and is of unknown cause (idiopathic). It is characterised by akinesia, a flexed posture, rigidity and a resting tremor. The pathological hallmark of Parkinson's disease is degeneration of the dopaminergic neurones of the pars compacta of the substantia nigra, and depletion of striatal dopamine levels (Fig. 11.8). The most effective treatment currently available for the condition is administration of levodopa (L-DOPA), the immediate metabolic precursor of dopamine, or dopamine receptor agonists. Levodopa is converted to dopamine and restores normal striatal function, a strategy which can often be used to minimise symptoms for many years.

Huntington's disease is a degenerative disease, inherited in an autosomal dominant manner and characterised by chorea and progressive dementia. Pathologically, there is progressive degeneration of the striatum and cerebral cortex. **Hepatolenticular degeneration (Wilson's disease)** is an inherited disorder (autosomal recessive) of copper metabolism. Basal ganglia changes lead to choreo-athetosis and progressive dementia in childhood and youth. **Sydenham's chorea** is now rare but was formerly a common manifestation of rheumatic fever in young females, causing abnormal behaviour and generalised chorea (**St. Vitus' dance**).

Levodopa-induced dyskinesia is a complication of the long-term treatment of Parkinson's disease with levodopa, and **tardive dyskinesia** is a long-term complication of the treatment of schizophrenia with neuroleptic drugs. **Hemiballism** is a rare condition characterised by violent choreiform movements of the limbs on one side of the body. It is caused by a lesion, usually of cerebrovascular origin, of the contralateral subthalamic nucleus. **Dystonia** may arise as an inherited disorder of children and is usually generalised. In adults, focal or segmental dystonias affect the arm and hand (writer's cramp), leg, neck (torticollis) or face and mouth (orofacial dyskinesia).

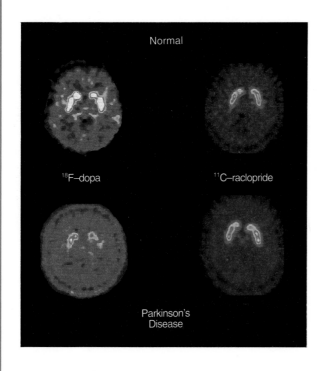

Fig. 11.8 **Four Positron Emission Tomography (PET) scans, representing horizonal sections through the brain (anterior towards the top in each case) at the level of the striatum.**
The top scans are from a normal individual and the bottom ones from a patient with Parkinson's disease. The scans on the left were made using the tracer ^{18}F-dopa. This is taken up by intact dopaminergic nerve terminals and, therefore, acts as an index of the integrity of the nigrostriatal pathway. Note the reduced labelling in the striatum of the parkinsonian patient. The scans on the right were made using the tracer ^{11}C-raclopride. This binds to dopamine receptors located on striatal neurones which receive input from the nigrostriatal pathway. Note that these receptors remain intact in the parkinsonian patient. (Courtesy of Professor D. J. Brooks, Consultant Neurologist, MRC Cyclotron Unit, Hammersmith Hospital, London.)

Visual system

Vision is the most highly developed and versatile of all the sensory modalities and, arguably, the one on which man is most dependent. The optic nerve and retina develop from the prosencephalic primary brain vesicle and thus are regarded as an outgrowth of the brain itself. Vision commences with the formation of an image of the external world on the photoreceptive **retina**. The retina encodes visual information in the discharge of neurones which project to the brain in the **optic nerve**. Fibres of the optic nerve undergo hemidecussation in the **optic chiasma** and project to the lateral geniculate nucleus of the thalamus. Thalamocortical neurones in turn project to the primary visual cortex of the occipital lobe where visual perception occurs.

THE EYE (Fig. 12.1)

The eyeball or globe is approximately spherical in shape. Near its posterior pole emerges the optic nerve. The eyeball may be considered to consist of three concentric layers of tissue, the outermost of which is tough, fibrous and protective. Over most of the globe it forms an opaque, white coat, the **sclera**, to which are attached the extraocular muscles. Over the anterior pole of the globe it forms the transparent **cornea**, through which light enters the eye.

Near to the anterior margin of the sclera, two rings of smooth muscle extend into the lumen of the eyeball (Fig. 12.2). The most anterior of these is the **iris**, whose central aperture is the **pupil** through which light is admitted to the posterior part of the eye. Some of the muscle fibres of the iris are arranged in a circular fashion whilst others are oriented radially. They are under the control of the autonomic nervous system. Circular fibres are innervated by parasympathetic neurones which act to constrict the pupil and reduce the

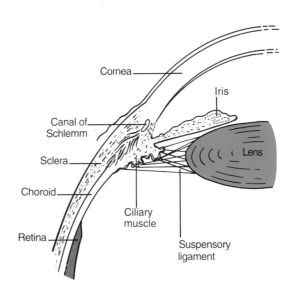

Fig. 12.1 **Schematic drawing of a horizontal section through the right eyeball**.

Fig. 12.2 **Schematic drawing of the sclerocorneal junction of the eyeball**.

amount of light falling upon the retina (see p. 74). Radial fibres are innervated by sympathetic neurones to dilate the pupil.

Behind the iris lies the **ciliary body**, containing **ciliary muscle** which receives innervation from the parasympathetic nervous system. The central aperture within the annulus of the ciliary body is occupied by the transparent, biconvex **lens** which focuses light upon the retina. The lens is held in place by a **suspensory ligament** which is attached to the peripheral margin of the lens and to the ciliary body. Contraction of the ciliary muscle alters the shape and, thus, the focusing power (focal length) of the lens, a process known as accommodation. The lens and suspensory ligament divide the lumen of the eyeball into an anterior and posterior part. The anterior part, in front of the lens, contains a thin, watery fluid, known as **aqueous humour**, which is continuously secreted from the ciliary body. Likewise, it is reabsorbed into the ciliary body where it accumulates in a small duct, the **canal of Schlemm**, through which it is returned to the venous system. The posterior part of the globe contains a gelatinous material known as **vitreous humour**. Behind the ciliary body, the inner surface of the sclera is lined by the **choroid**, whose cells contain dark pigment which absorbs light and thus reduces reflection within the eye. Lining the inner surface of the choroid is the photoreceptive retina.

Light passes from objects in the field of vision (**visual field**), through the narrow aperture of the pupil, to subtend an image upon the retina. An object in the visual field, upon which attention is focused, subtends

an image which is centred near the posterior pole of the eye, along the line of the **visual axis** (Fig. 12.1). At this point, which is known as the **fovea centralis**, and the surrounding 1 cm, which is known as the **macula lutea**, the retina is specially modified for maximal visual acuity (resolving power). The basic optical properties of the eye, which may be likened to those of a pin-hole camera, dictate that the image so formed is inverted in both lateral and vertical dimensions (Fig. 12.3). Furthermore, objects which lie in the left half of the visual field form an image upon the nasal (right) half of the left retina and the temporal (right) half of the right retina, and vice versa. Medial to the macula is a region where retinal axons accumulate to leave the eye in the optic nerve. This is known as the **optic disc**. Photoreceptors are absent from this region which is also referred to as the **blind spot**.

RETINA (Fig. 12.4)

The retina consists of a non-neural and a neural portion. The non-neural part is represented by the **pigment epithelium**, a single layer of light-absorbing, pigmented cells lying adjacent to the choroid. The neural part of the retina contains photoreceptors and neurones as well as neuroglia and a rich capillary network. The photoreceptive cells lie deepest within the retina and interdigitate with the pigment epithelium. Light entering the eye thus passes through, and is refracted and partially absorbed by, these additional elements before reaching the photoreceptors. By means of a series of photochemical reactions and physicochemical

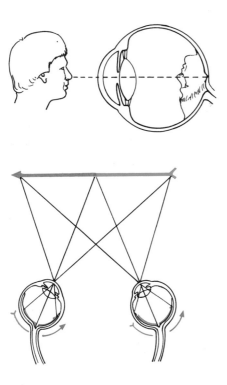

Fig. 12.3 **The representation of the visual field upon the retinae.**

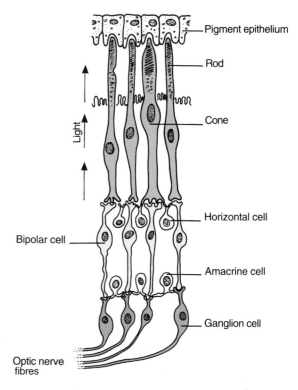

Fig. 12.4 **Schematic drawing showing the cellular organisation of the retina.**

changes, retinal photoreceptors transduce light energy into electrical energy (changes in membrane potential). Retinal photoreceptors are of two types, **rods** and **cones**, of which the rods are about 20 times more numerous. These cells share many structural similarities but have important functional distinctions. Rods are exquisitely sensitive to light. They are, thus, particularly important for vision in dim lighting conditions. Cones are responsible for colour vision and, because of their arrangement and neuronal connections, they confer high visual acuity.

Rods and cones are heterogeneously distributed across the retina. Rods greatly predominate in the peripheral parts of the retina but their relative numbers decrease towards the macula, where cones are more abundant. At the fovea only cones are present. Furthermore, at the fovea the neurones and capillaries, through which light has to pass to reach the photoreceptors, are displaced so that the cones are directly exposed to light. This combination provides for maximal visual acuity.

In addition to photoreceptive cells, the retina contains both the first- and second-order neurones of the visual pathway (Fig. 12.4). The first-order neurone, or **bipolar cell**, lies entirely within the retina whilst the axon of the second-order neurone, or **ganglion cell**, constitutes the optic nerve. Information is transferred from photoreceptors to bipolar cells and, thence, to ganglion cells with greater convergence for rods than for cones. The retina also contains interneurones known as horizontal cells and amacrine cells. These modulate transmission between photoreceptors and bipolar cells and between bipolar cells and ganglion cells, respectively.

The eye

- Objects in one lateral half of the visual field form images on the nasal half of the ipsilateral retina and the temporal half of the contralateral retina.
- The retina contains photoreceptors (rods and cones), first-order sensory neurones (bipolar cells) and second-order neurones (ganglion cells).
- The axons of retinal ganglion cells accumulate at the optic disc (blind spot) and pass into the optic nerve.

THE CENTRAL VISUAL PATHWAY (Fig. 12.5)

The axons of retinal ganglion cells assemble at the optic disc and pass into the optic nerve which enters the cranial cavity through the optic canal. The two optic nerves converge to form the **optic chiasma** on the base of the brain. The chiasma lies immediately rostral to the tuber cinereum of the hypothalamus and between the terminating internal carotid arteries. In the chiasma, axons derived from the nasal halves of the two retinae decussate and pass into the contralateral **optic tract**, whilst those from the temporal hemiretinae remain ipsilateral. The optic tracts diverge away from the chiasma and pass round the cerebral peduncle to terminate mainly in the lateral geniculate nucleus (within the lateral geniculate body) of the thalamus. A relatively small number of fibres leave the optic nerve, before reaching the lateral geniculate nucleus, to terminate in the **pretectal area** and the superior colliculus. These fibres are involved in mediation of the pupillary light reflex (see p. 74). From the lateral geniculate nucleus, third-order thalamocortical neurones project through the retrolenticular part of the internal capsule forming the **optic radiation**, which terminates in the primary visual cortex of the occipital lobe. The primary visual cortex is located predominantly on the medial surface of the hemisphere in the region above and below the calcarine sulcus. Surrounding this area the rest of the occipital lobe constitutes the visual association cortex. It is concerned with interpretation of visual images, recognition, depth perception and colour vision.

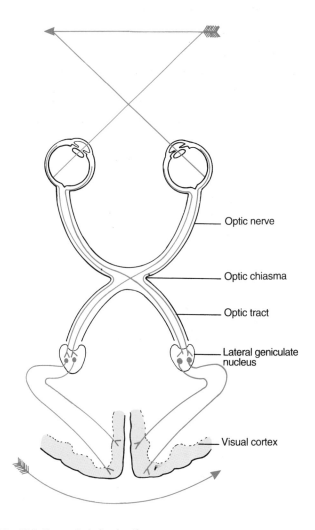

Optic nerve

Optic chiasma

Optic tract

Lateral geniculate nucleus

Visual cortex

Fig. 12.5 **The central visual pathway**.

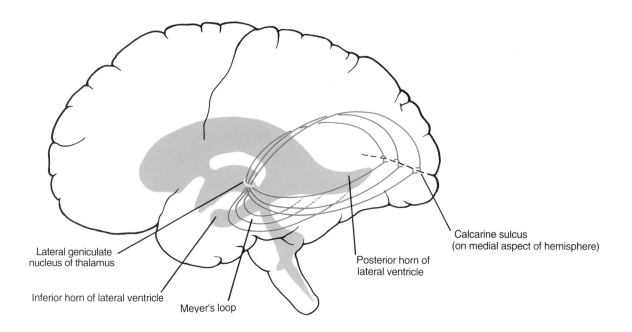

Fig. 12.6 **The course taken by thalamocortical fibres projecting from the lateral geniculate nucleus to the primary visual cortex.**

There is a precise point-to-point relationship between the retina and the visual cortex. Because of the importance of the macula in vision, it is represented by disproportionately large volumes (relative to its size) of the lateral geniculate nucleus and the visual cortex. Within the visual cortex the macula is represented most posteriorly, in the region of the occipital pole.

As previously noted, objects in either half (left or right) of the visual field produce images upon the nasal hemiretina of the ipsilateral eye and the temporal hemiretina of the contralateral eye (Fig. 12.5). Each optic nerve, thus, carries information concerning both halves of the visual field. Due to the decussation of fibres from the nasal hemiretinae at the optic chiasma, however, each optic tract, lateral geniculate nucleus and visual cortex receives information relating only to the contralateral half of the visual field. This combination of the images from both eyes is necessary for stereoscopic vision (depth perception). The upper half of the visual field forms images upon the lower halves of the retinae, the lower visual field upon the upper hemiretinae. As thalamocortical fibres leave the lateral geniculate nucleus they pass around the lateral ventricle, those representing the lower part of the visual field coursing superiorly to terminate in the visual cortex above the calcarine sulcus. Those which represent the upper part of the visual field sweep into the temporal lobe (**Meyer's loop**, Fig. 12.6) before terminating below the calcarine sulcus.

The visual field can be considered (Fig. 12.7) as comprising four quadrants (left\right, upper\lower) each projecting to its own quadrant of the primary visual cortex (left\right, above\below the calcarine sulcus).

There is both lateral and vertical inversion in the projection of the visual field upon the visual cortex such that, for example, the upper left quadrant of the visual field is represented in the lower right quadrant of the visual cortex.

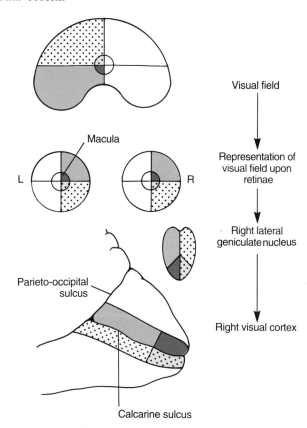

Fig. 12.7 **Diagram showing the representation of the left half of the visual field at the various levels of the visual pathway.**

The central visual pathway

- At the optic chiasma, axons from the nasal halves of the two retinae decussate and pass into the contralateral optic tract.
- The optic tract contains axons which carry information relating to the contralateral half of the field of vision.
- Optic tract fibres end in the lateral geniculate nucleus of the thalamus.
- Third-order visual fibres from the lateral geniculate nucleus pass through the retrolenticular part of the internal capsule and the visual radiations to terminate in the primary visual cortex.
- The primary visual cortex is located above and below the calcarine sulcus of the occipital lobe.
- The rest of the occipital lobe constitutes the visual association area.

Visual field deficits

Disease of the eyeball (cataract, intraocular haemorrhage, retinal detachment) and disease of the optic nerve (multiple sclerosis and optic nerve tumours) lead to loss of vision in the affected eye (**monocular blindness**). Compression of the optic chiasm by an adjacent pituitary tumour leads to **bitemporal hemianopia**. Vascular and neoplastic lesions of the optic tract, optic radiation or occipital cortex produce a contralateral **homonymous hemianopia** (Fig. 12.8).

Retinitis pigmentosa is an inherited metabolic disorder of the photoreceptor and retinal pigment epithelial cells. There is progressive night blindness, peripheral visual field constriction and pigmentation of the retina visible on ophthalmoscopy.

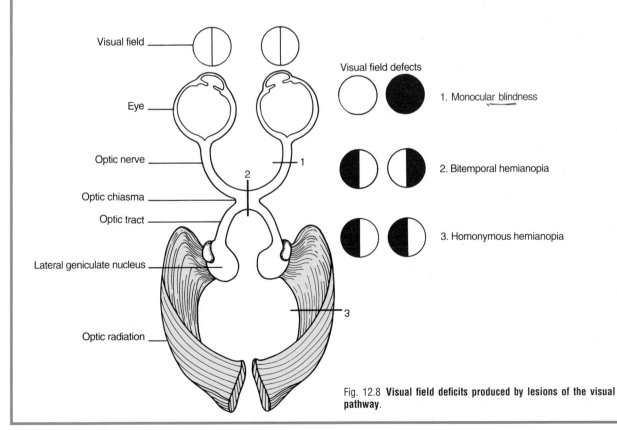

Fig. 12.8 **Visual field deficits produced by lesions of the visual pathway**.

Hypothalamus, limbic system and olfactory system

In order to survive, there must be continual adaptations to preserve the internal homeostasis (internal milieu) of the organism. Interoceptor signals from the internal organs and body fluids initiate homeostatic responses so that the internal physical and chemical environment remains balanced and stable. The hypothalamus is the structure responsible for this task.

Exteroceptive information from the environment dictates behavioural responses of the whole organism in order to achieve individual homeostasis within the physical and social environment. Behaviour may be relatively simple and stereotyped in lower animals and directed to satisfying the drives of thirst, hunger, sex and defence in instinctive repertoires. The limbic system, which is strongly connected to the hypothalamus, is essential for this adaptive behaviour, which includes the ability to learn new responses based on previous experience (memory). The complex and non-stereotyped behaviour of man is an attempt to preserve the individual within the physical landscape but also within a changing social environment (individual homeostasis). The association areas of the neocortex are capable of analysing exteroceptive information from the environment and other individuals, enabling adaptive personal and social responses. These phylogenetically more recent structures are partly connected to the limbic system.

Thus in a hierarchical fashion the hypothalamus, limbic system and association neocortex act as interfaces between the internal structure of the individual and his environment. A reminder of this evolutionary ascent in man is the olfactory system, vital to sensing the environment in lower animals, overwhelmed by the visuospatial dominance of man, and intimately related to the limbic system.

HYPOTHALAMUS

The hypothalamus is able to integrate interoceptive signals from internal organs and fluid-filled cavities and make appropriate adjustments to the internal milieu by virtue of its input and output systems.

The hypothalamic input is circulatory and neural in origin. In the circulating blood come physical (temperature, osmolality), chemical (blood glucose, acid–base state) and hormonal signals of the state of the organism, its growth and development and its readiness for action (sex, suckling, defence). Neural signals come from two sources. Firstly, the nucleus solitarius of the medulla projects to the hypothalamus and conveys information collected by the autonomic nervous system, concerning the pressure within the smooth muscled walls of organs (baroreceptors) and the chemical constituents of the fluid-filled cavities (chemoreceptors). Secondly, the state of neural arousal is communicated by two structures in the midbrain: the reticular formation via direct and indirect (via thalamus) routes, and the monoaminergic nuclei, via the medial forebrain bundle.

The hypothalamus is capable of generating responses to these stimuli by circulatory and neural means. An intimate relationship to the pituitary gland and privileged access to the circulation (portal system) confers the role of 'orchestrator of the endocrine system' on the hypothalamus, as it directs hormonal synthesis and release. The neural output of the hypothalamus is twofold. Firstly, the autonomic nervous system projects to and controls internal organs, outside conscious control (and, hence, autonomous). Secondly, the hypothalamus is capable of initiating appropriate motor behavioural repertoires of an instinctive kind, through its connections with the limbic system and limbic part of the corpus striatum (the nucleus accumbens). Its interconnections with the reticular formation also are capable of influencing the state of wakefulness and sleep.

The hypothalamus has the capability of influencing or overriding more complex adaptive behaviour because of its close links with two important structures: the limbic system and the association cortex of the frontal lobe (orbital part).

TOPOGRAPHICAL ANATOMY OF THE HYPOTHALAMUS

The hypothalamus is the most ventral part of the diencephalon, lying beneath the thalamus and ventromedial to the subthalamus. It forms the floor and the lower part of the lateral wall of the third ventricle, below the hypothalamic sulcus (Fig. 9.2). On the base of the brain, parts of the hypothalamus can be seen occupying the small area circumscribed by the crura cerebri, optic chiasma and optic tracts (Fig. 9.1). Between the rostral limits of the two crura cerebri, on either side of the middle, lie two distinct, rounded eminences, the **mammillary bodies**, which contain the **mammillary nuclei**. In the midline, immediately caudal to the optic chiasma, lies a small elevated area known as the **tuber cinereum**, from the apex of which extends the thin **infundibulum** (**infundibular process**), or **pituitary stalk**. In life this bears the **pituitary gland** (**hypophysis**), a pea-sized structure which lies within the sella turcica of the sphenoid bone. The pituitary gland consists of two major, cytologically distinct, parts: the

posterior pituitary or **neurohypophysis** and the anterior pituitary or **adenohypophysis** (see Figs 13.2 and 13.3). The posterior pituitary is a neuronal structure, being an expansion of the distal part of the infundibular process. The anterior pituitary is not neural in origin. The two parts are, however, closely linked by the **pituitary** (hypophyseal) **portal system** of vessels (see Fig. 13.3), which are derived from the superior hypophyseal artery. Releasing factors, which are synthesised in the hypothalamus, pass to the adenohypophysis through these vessels to control the release of anterior pituitary hormones.

HYPOTHALAMIC NUCLEI

The hypothalamus consists of many nuclear divisions, only some of which will be described (Figs 13.1 and 11.5). The region lying medial and ventral to the structures of the subthalamus is known as the **lateral hypothalamus**. It is traversed longitudinally by many fibres including the medial forebrain bundle. The lateral hypothalamic area is important in the control of food and water intake and is, in part, equivalent to the physiologically-defined feeding centre. Lateral hypothalamic lesions cause aphagia and adipsia.

The medial region of the hypothalamus contains various nuclei, only some of which have well defined functions. Anteriorly lie the supraoptic, paraventricular and suprachiasmatic nuclei. The supraoptic and paraventricular nuclei both produce systemically-acting hormones, which are released from the posterior pituitary into the general circulation. The **supraoptic nu-**

Fig. 13.1 **A sagittal section of the diencephalon**.
The diagram shows the medial aspect of the hypothalamus. The approximate location of some of the principal hypothalamic nuclei are shown.

cleus produces vasopressin (antidiuretic hormone) which increases water reabsorption by the kidney. The **paraventricular nucleus** synthesises oxytocin. In the female, activation of the paraventricular nucleus, and release of hormone, is induced by suckling. This stimulates milk production by the mammary gland and causes contraction of uterine muscle.

The axons of cells in the supraoptic and paraventricular nuclei pass to the neurohypophysis in the hypothalamohypophyseal tract (Fig. 13.2). The neuroendocrine products are transported in this tract to the neurohypophysis where they are released into the capillary bed and, thus, reach the general circulation.

The supraoptic nucleus contains osmosensitive neurones whose activity is affected by the osmolality of circulating blood. An increase in osmolality activates the neurones and causes release of vasopressin. This acts upon the kidney tubules to increase water reabsorption, thus maintaining water homeostasis.

The hypothalamus also synthesises releasing factors and release-inhibiting factors which control the release of hormones by the adenohypophysis. The adenohypophysis produces: adrenocorticotrophic hormone (ACTH), luteinising hormone (LH), follicle stimulating hormone (FSH), thyroid stimulating hormone (TSH), growth hormone and prolactin—which are released into the general circulation. The factors which control them are released from the terminals of hypothalamic neurones into the capillary bed of the pituitary portal system (Fig. 13.3). These vessels, which are intrinsic to the hypophyseal stalk, convey the released agents to the adenohypophysis where they act

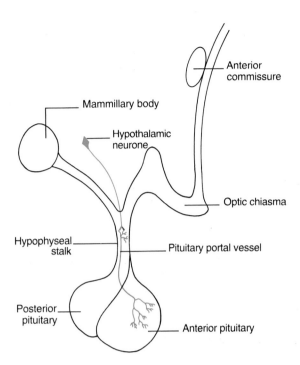

Fig. 13.3 **Pituitary portal system linking anterior and posterior parts of the pituitary gland**.

upon the hormone secreting cells. The synthesis of hypothalamic releasing factors is under feedback regulation by hormones produced by target organs.

The **suprachiasmatic nucleus** is concerned with the control of diurnal rhythms and the sleep\waking cycle. It receives some afferent fibres direct from the retina.

More caudally, dorsomedial and ventromedial nuclei lie deep to the lateral wall of the third ventricle. The **ventromedial nucleus**, like the lateral hypothalamus, is concerned with the control of food and fluid intake. The ventromedial nucleus is equated with the physiologically-defined satiety centre and lesions of this region cause abnormally increased food intake. In the most caudal part of the hypothalamus lie the pos-

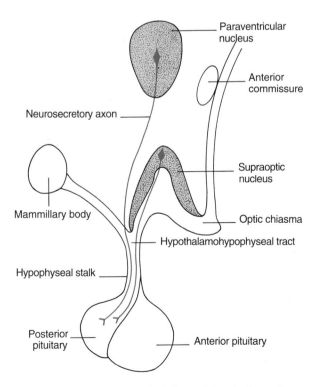

Fig. 13.2 **Supraoptic and paraventricular nuclei projecting to the posterior pituitary via the hypothalamohypophyseal tract**.

Tumours of the hypothalamus and pituitary gland

Tumours and other diseases of the hypothalamus and associated pituitary gland lead to under- or overproduction of circulating hormones. These, in turn, produce disorders of growth (**dwarfism**, **gigantism** and **acromegaly**), sexual function (**precocious puberty**, **hypogonadism**), body water control (**diabetes insipidus** and **pathological drinking**), eating (**obesity** and **bulimia**) and adrenal cortical control (**Cushing's disease** and **adrenal insufficiency**). Since the pituitary gland is closely adjacent to the optic chiasma, tumours of the gland (**pituitary adenomas**) may lead to bitemporal visual field loss.

terior nucleus and the **medial mammillary nucleus**, the latter being located within the mammillary body. The mammillary body is part of the limbic system, receiving afferents from the hippocampus and projecting to the anterior nuclei of the thalamus and the brain stem.

The hypothalamus is the brain centre for regulation of the autonomic nervous system. Generally, activation of the posterior hypothalamic domain is associated with sympathetic responses, whereas activation of the anterior hypothalamus is associated with parasympathetic activity.

Hypothalamus

- The hypothalamus is part of the diencephalon.
- The hypothalamus has autonomic, neuroendocrine and limbic functions and is involved in the coordination of homeostatic mechanisms.
- Through the infundibular process, the hypothalamus is connected to the pituitary gland.
- The hypothalamus produces hormones which are released from the posterior pituitary and also releasing factors which control the release of hormones from the anterior pituitary.
- The supraoptic nucleus of the hypothalamus produces vasopressin.
- The paraventricular nucleus produces oxytocin.
- Vasopressin and oxytocin are transported to the posterior pituitary in the hypothalamohypophyseal tract.
- The anterior pituitary produces: adrenocorticotrophic hormone, luteinising hormone, follicle stimulating hormone, thyroid stimulating hormone, growth hormone and prolactin. Factors which control their secretion are released into the pituitary portal system of the pituitary stalk and carried to the anterior pituitary.
- The lateral hypothalamus and the ventromedial nucleus regulate eating and drinking.

LIMBIC SYSTEM

The limbic system earns its title from its position on the medial rim of the brain (le grand lobe limbique). It consists of a number of structures with complex and often looped connections which all ultimately project into the hypothalamus (Fig. 13.4). The powerful input to the limbic system from the neocortical association areas links complex 'goal directed' behaviour to more primitive instinctual behaviour and internal homeostasis in a cascade of neural connections (Figs 13.5 and 13.6). An oversimplified view would conceive of information from the outside world collected in modality specific ways (e.g. vision, hearing and touch) and refined in the parietal–occipital association areas (perceptuospatial function). This information is then conveyed to the frontal association areas involved in planned behaviour

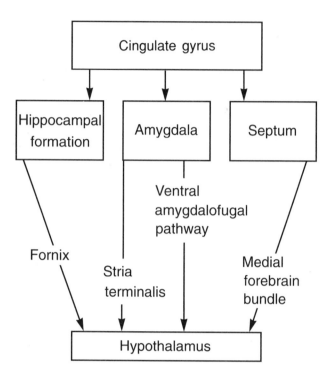

Fig. 13.4 **The principal parts of the limbic system and their relationship with the hypothalamus**.

(regulation) and also to the inferior temporal association areas, where information can reach supramodal status and meaning (semantic processing). Entry of information into the limbic system is either directly, to the amygdala, or indirectly to the hippocampal formation, via the entorhinal area. The amygdala appears to provide an affective connotation to experience and especially that relevant to social stimuli. Perhaps affect is an evolutionary development from more primitive 'feelings', derived from the sensory autonomic input from bodily organs into the hypothalamus. The informational flow into the hippocampal formation permits a link to previous experience since the hippocampal formation is essential to remembering and learning (memory).

The limbic system is able to influence motor responses, appropriate to its informational analyses, through projections to the nucleus accumbens, which forms part of the basal ganglia.

AMYGDALA

The amygdala lies near the temporal pole, between the inferior horn of the lateral ventricle and the lentiform nucleus (Fig. 10.8). It receives afferents from the inferior temporal association cortex, the septum and the olfactory tract. In addition it receives catecholamine and 5-HT-containing projections from the brain stem in the medial forebrain bundle. The principal efferent projection from the amygdala is the stria terminalis

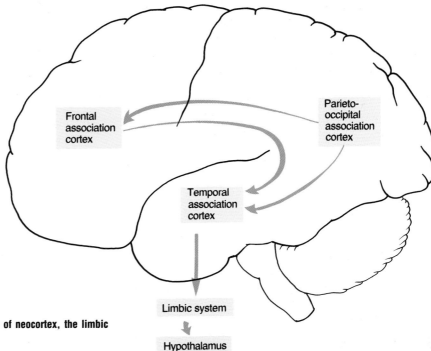

Fig. 13.5 **The link between associative areas of neocortex, the limbic system and the hypothalamus**.

Fig. 13.6 **The interconnections between associative neocortical regions and the component parts of the limbic system**.

which runs in the wall of the lateral ventricle, following the curvature of the caudate nucleus, to terminate ultimately in the hypothalamus. The ventral amygdalofugal path also projects to the hypothalamus.

SEPTUM

The septum, or septal region, lies beneath the rostral part of the corpus callosum. It interconnects with the amygdala and projects to the hypothalamus via the medial forebrain bundle. The septum also connects to the monoaminergic nuclei in the brain stem. It does so via fibres which project to the **habenular nuclei** of the diencephalon and constitute the **stria medullaris thalami**. The habenular nuclei in turn project, via the fasciculus retroflexus, to the **interpeduncular nuclei** which project to the brain stem as well as the hypothalamus. Thus two major pathways link the septum, hypothalamus and the monoaminergic nuclei of the brain stem.

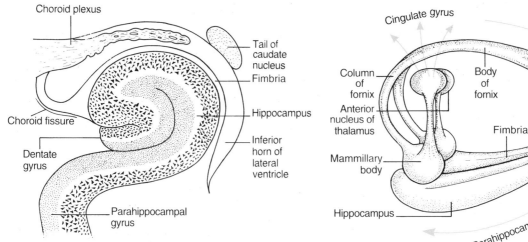

Fig. 13.7 **Transverse section through the hippocampus and inferior horn of the lateral ventricle.**

Fig. 13.8 **The interconnection of limbic structures which constitute the Papez circuit.**

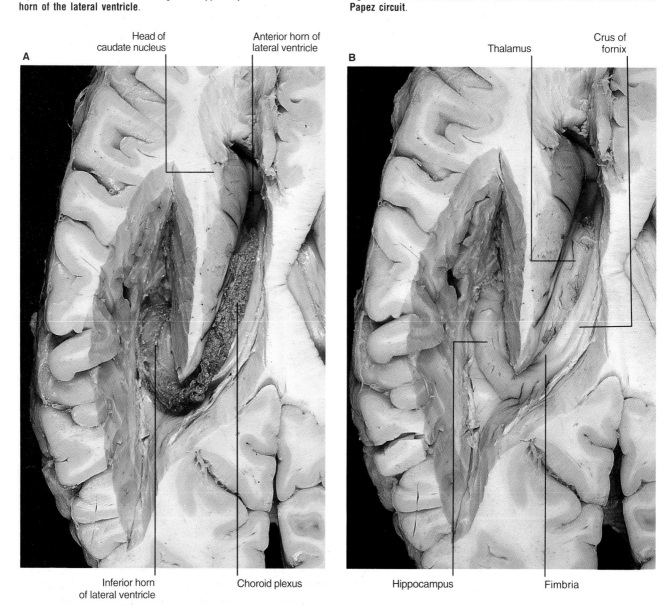

Fig. 13.9 **The hippocampus–fimbria–fornix system.**
The brain is viewed from above. The cerebral cortex and white matter, including the corpus callosum, have been removed to reveal the lateral ventricle and its contents. (**A**) Choroid plexus of lateral ventricle intact; (**B**) choroid plexus removed.

HIPPOCAMPAL FORMATION

The hippocampal formation consists of the hippocampus itself, the dentate gyrus and parts of the parahippocampal gyrus. The **hippocampus** is formed by an infolding of the inferomedial part of the temporal lobe into the lateral ventricle, along the line of the choroid fissure (Fig. 13.7 and Figs 10.8–10.12). The **dentate gyrus** lies between the parahippocampal gyrus and the hippocampus.

The hippocampal formation receives afferents principally from the inferior temporal cortex, via the entorhinal area of the temporal lobe. It also receives fibres from the contralateral entorhinal area and hippocampus via the fornix system and hippocampal commissure. The principal efferent pathway from the hippocampus is the **fornix** (Figs 9.2, 10.2 and 10.7–10.12). The fornix is a prominent C-shaped fascicle of fibres which links the hippocampus with the mammillary body of the hypothalamus (Fig. 13.8). Efferent fibres converge on the ventricular surface of the hippocampus as the **fimbria**. This passes posteriorly and superiorly to become continuous with the crus of the fornix, which then curves forward beneath the splenium of the corpus callosum. The two crura unite in the midline, beneath the corpus callosum, to form the body of the fornix and some fibres cross to the opposite side through the small hippocampal commissure. As it passes forwards beneath the corpus callosum, the body of the fornix divides into two columns which then curve downwards forming the anterior border of the interventricular foramen and enter the hypothalamus where the majority of fibres terminate in the mammillary body. The mammillary body in turn projects to the anterior nuclear group of the thalamus via the mammillothalamic tract and to the brain stem via the mammillotegmental tract. The anterior nuclei of the thalamus have major connections with the cingulate gyrus.

CINGULATE GYRUS

The cingulate gyrus and the **parahippocampal gyrus** are in continuity with one another around the splenium of the corpus callosum (Fig. 13.10). The cingulate gyrus projects to the parahippocampal gyrus via the fibres of the cingulum (see Ch. 10). The principal structures of the limbic system are thus linked by a series of connections which constitute the **Papez circuit** (Fig. 13.8).

Limbic system

- The amygdala is located near to the temporal pole. It receives projections from the olfactory system and the temporal cortex and has reciprocal connections with the septum.
- The hippocampal formation is made up of the hippocampus, dentate gyrus and parahippocampal gyrus of the temporal lobe. It receives fibres from the entorhinal cortex and projects via the fornix to the mammillary body of the hypothalamus.
- The principal components of the limbic system are interconnected in the Papez circuit.

Limbic lobe disorders

Alcohol abuse in a setting of dietary deficiency of thiamine leads to capillary haemorrhages in the upper brain stem and limbic structures. The patient falls into confusion and coma (**Wernicke's encephalopathy**). Partial recovery may occur with failure to remember previous experience (retrograde amnesia) or to learn new facts (anterograde amnesia). This is known as **Korsakoff's psychosis**. A similar amnesic syndrome occurs when bilateral, surgical temporal lobectomy incorporates the hippocampal formations.

Temporal lobe or **complex partial seizures** arising close to the amygdala and hippocampi can lead to complex experiences of smell, mood and memory. The states of disordered thinking, hallucinations and strange or violent behaviour can mimic schizophrenia. Surgical ablation of the amygdala has eliminated uncontrollable rage reactions in some psychotic patients.

OLFACTORY SYSTEM

Olfactory receptors are specialised, ciliated nerve cells which lie in the olfactory epithelium of the nasal cavity. Their axons assemble into numerous small fascicles (the true olfactory nerves), which enter the cranial cavity through the foramina of the **cribriform plate** of the ethmoid bone (Fig. 4.1) and then attach to the **olfactory bulb** on the inferior surface of the frontal lobe

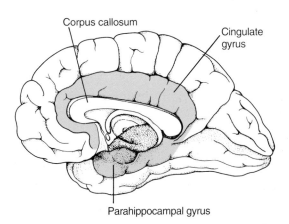

Corpus callosum

Cingulate gyrus

Parahippocampal gyrus

Fig. 13.10 **Medial aspect of the cerebral hemisphere showing the relationship between the cingulate gyrus and parahippocampal gyrus.**

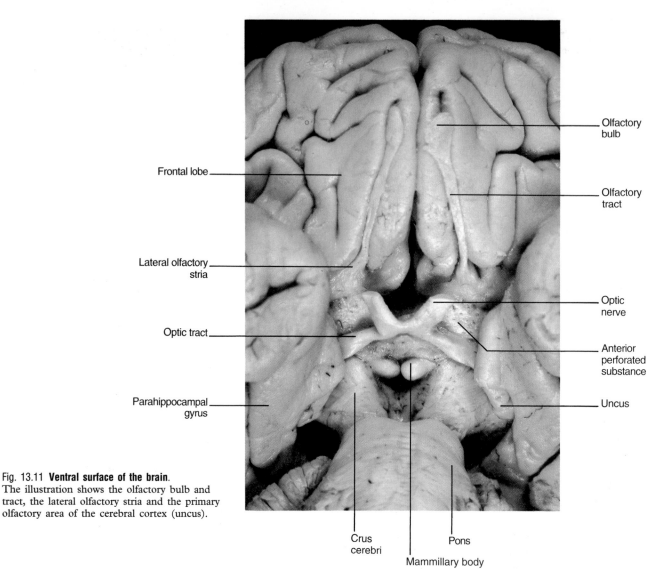

Frontal lobe

Lateral olfactory stria

Optic tract

Parahippocampal gyrus

Olfactory bulb

Olfactory tract

Optic nerve

Anterior perforated substance

Uncus

Crus cerebri

Pons

Mammillary body

Fig. 13.11 **Ventral surface of the brain.** The illustration shows the olfactory bulb and tract, the lateral olfactory stria and the primary olfactory area of the cerebral cortex (uncus).

(Fig. 13.11 and Fig. 7.1). Preliminary processing of olfactory information occurs within the olfactory bulb, which contains interneurones and large **mitral cells** whose axons leave the bulb in the olfactory tract.

The olfactory tract passes backwards on the basal surface of the frontal lobe and, just before reaching the level of the optic chiasma, the majority of olfactory tract fibres are deflected laterally, in the **lateral olfactory stria** (Fig. 13.11). These fibres pass into the depths of the lateral fissure which they cross to reach the temporal lobe. They terminate mainly in the **primary olfactory cortex** of the **uncus** (Fig. 13.11 and Fig. 10.2), on the inferomedial aspect of the temporal lobe, and in the subadjacent amygdala. Adjacent to the uncus, the anterior part of the parahippocampal gyrus, or entorhinal area, constitutes the olfactory association cortex. The primary and association cortices are also collectively referred to as the pyriform cortex and are responsible for the appreciation of olfactory stimuli. The olfactory projection is unique among the sensory systems in that it consists of a sequence of only two neurones between the sensory receptors and cerebral cortex and does not project via the thalamus.

Anosmia

Anosmia follows damage to the olfactory nerves. There is loss, not only of the sense of smell, but of the flavour of foods. However, elementary aspects of taste, e.g. sweet, salt, bitter and sour are preserved. Anosmia frequently follows head trauma and can occur when tumours of the meninges (**meningiomas**) invade the olfactory nerves.

Olfactory system

- Olfactory nerve fibres terminate in the olfactory bulb.
- Second-order fibres run in the olfactory tract and terminate in the primary olfactory cortex of the uncus in the temporal lobe.
- Adjacent to this, the anterior part of the parahippocampal gyrus, or entorhinal cortex, constitutes the olfactory association cortex.

Autonomic nervous system

The term autonomic nervous system is used to encompass those nerve cells, located within both the central and peripheral nervous systems, which are concerned with the innervation and control of visceral organs, smooth muscle and secretory glands. The principal function of the autonomic nervous system is broadly described as homeostasis of the internal environment. This is achieved by regulation of cardiovascular, respiratory, digestive, excretory and thermoregulatory mechanisms, which occurs automatically and with relatively little volitional control.

Autonomic afferent and efferent fibres enter and leave the central nervous system through spinal and cranial nerves. Within the spinal cord and brain stem they establish interconnections through which autonomic reflexes are mediated. Afferent fibres also establish connections with ascending neurones through which conscious awareness of visceral function is achieved. Changes in the internal and external environment, and emotional factors, profoundly influence autonomic activity, most notably via descending connections from the hypothalamus. Autonomic efferent neurones differ from those of the somatic nervous system in that there is a sequence of two neurones between the CNS and the innervated structure (Fig. 14.1). The cell body of the first neurone is located in the spinal cord or brain stem whilst that of the second neurone is located peripherally in an **autonomic ganglion**. The first neurone is referred to as the **preganglionic neurone** and the second as the **postganglionic neurone**.

The efferent neurones of the autonomic nervous system fall into two distinct anatomical and functional groups or divisions, namely, **sympathetic** and **parasympathetic**. Many, though not all, structures which receive autonomic fibres are dually innervated by both sympathetic and parasympathetic systems. These exercise antagonistic effects upon the innervated structure.

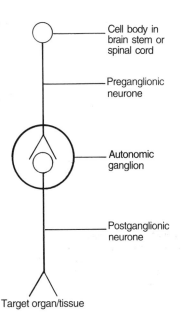

Fig. 14.1 **Basic organisation of the autonomic nervous system into preganglionic and postganglionic neurones.**
In the sympathetic division, ganglia constitute the sympathetic chain. Preganglionic neurones, therefore, have relatively short axons whilst postganglionic fibres are relatively long. In the parasympathetic division, ganglia are located close to the target organ. Thus, preganglionic axons are long and postganglionic axons are short.

SYMPATHETIC DIVISION
(Figs 14.2 and 14.3)

Preganglionic sympathetic neurones are located exclusively in the thoracic and upper two or three lumbar segments of the spinal cord. They lie in the **lateral horn** of the spinal grey matter which is, therefore, only present at these levels (Figs 5.7 and 5.8). Preganglionic axons leave the cord in the ventral nerve root and join the spinal nerve. Postganglionic sympathetic neurones have their cell bodies in one of two locations, either the **sympathetic chain** of ganglia which lies alongside the vertebral column, or the plexuses (coeliac, superior

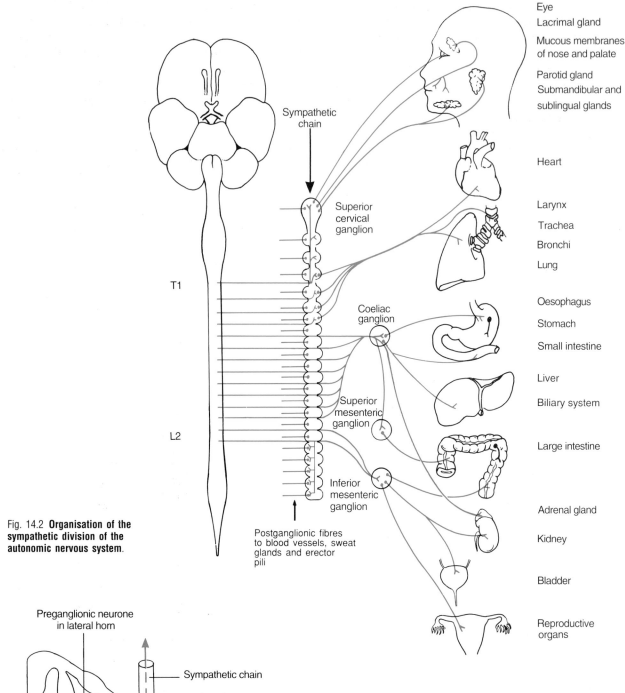

Eye
Lacrimal gland
Mucous membranes
of nose and palate
Parotid gland
Submandibular and
sublingual glands

Heart

Larynx
Trachea
Bronchi
Lung

Oesophagus
Stomach
Small intestine

Liver
Biliary system

Large intestine

Adrenal gland
Kidney

Bladder

Reproductive
organs

Sympathetic
chain

Superior
cervical
ganglion

Coeliac
ganglion

Superior
mesenteric
ganglion

Inferior
mesenteric
ganglion

T1

L2

Postganglionic fibres
to blood vessels, sweat
glands and erector
pili

Fig. 14.2 **Organisation of the
sympathetic division of the
autonomic nervous system**.

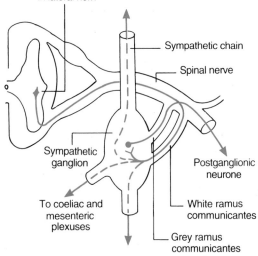

Preganglionic neurone
in lateral horn

Sympathetic chain

Spinal nerve

Sympathetic
ganglion

Postganglionic
neurone

To coeliac and
mesenteric
plexuses

White ramus
communicantes

Grey ramus
communicantes

Fig. 14.3 **Relationships between a typical thoracic spinal nerve and
the sympathetic chain**.

mesenteric, inferior mesenteric) which surround the main branches of the abdominal aorta. In order to reach either of these locations, preganglionic axons in the spinal nerve enter the sympathetic chain. Ganglia of the sympathetic chain are linked to those spinal nerves which contain sympathetic outflow by two small nerves, the **rami communicantes** (Fig. 14.3). Preganglionic fibres pass into the chain via the white ramus communicantes, so called because the fibres are myelinated.

Those fibres concerned with innervation of structures in the head and thorax terminate in synaptic contact with postganglionic cell bodies in the sympathetic chain. The postganglionic fibres return to the spinal nerve via the grey ramus communicantes, so called because the fibres are unmyelinated. Those preganglionic fibres concerned with innervation of pelvic and abdominal viscera pass uninterrupted through the sympathetic chain and travel to the plexuses where their corresponding postganglionic cells are located. The neurotransmitter released by preganglionic sympathetic neurones is acetylcholine. The transmitter of postganglionic sympathetic cells is generally noradrenaline, although the cells innervating sweat glands are cholinergic. The adrenal medulla is an exceptional organ in that it is directly innervated by preganglionic sympathetic neurons.

The effects of sympathetic nervous system activity are most apparent under conditions of stress, excitement or fear and are classically referred to as the 'flight or fight' response. The heart rate and blood pressure are increased. The bronchi are dilated to increase air flow to and from the lungs. Vasodilatation in skeletal muscles allows increased blood flow required for energetic activity whilst gastrointestinal blood flow and motility are decreased. Metabolic changes occur, such as an increase in blood glucose, to support high energy utilisation and sweating occurs to increase heat loss.

PARASYMPATHETIC DIVISION (Fig. 14.4)

Preganglionic parasympathetic neurones are located in the brain stem and the spinal cord. Within the brain stem such cells lie in cranial nerve nuclei associated

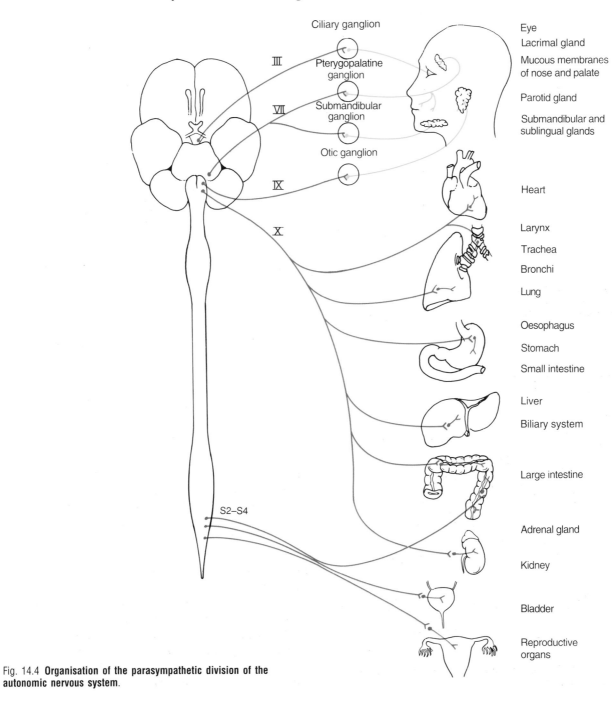

Fig. 14.4 **Organisation of the parasympathetic division of the autonomic nervous system**.

with the oculomotor, facial, glossopharyngeal and vagus nerves and provide innervation for structures of the head, thorax and abdomen. The parasympathetic components of these nerves are described in Chapter 7. Within the cord, preganglionic parasympathetic neurones lie in the second, third and fourth sacral segments and provide innervation for pelvic viscera. The cell bodies of postganglionic parasympathetic neurones lie in ganglia which are located close to the structure which they innervate. Within the alimentary canal these neurones contribute to the myenteric (Auerbach's) and submucosal (Meissner's) plexuses.

These plexuses are also referred to as the 'enteric nervous system'. Such a concept has arisen because the plexuses additionally contain afferent neurones and interneurones. The rich local interconnections of these cells are capable of sustaining the motility of the gastrointestinal tract in the absence of input from the central nervous system. Furthermore, these cells cannot simply be equated with the parasympathetic nervous system, since they are also known to receive synaptic input from postganglionic sympathetic neurones. The neurotransmitter released by both preganglionic and postganglionic parasympathetic neurones is acetylcholine.

Lesions of the sympathetic nervous system

Primary autonomic failure is a chronic degenerative disease of the nervous system and leads to fainting due to failure to control the heart rate and blood pressure (**postural syncope**), incontinence of urine and bowel, and impotence.

Horner's syndrome refers to drooping of the eyelid (ptosis), and constriction of the pupil (miosis) due to damage to the sympathetic nerves to the levator palpebrae superioris and the radial (pupillodilator) fibres of the iris. The sympathetic nerves may be damaged as they descend in the brain stem (by stroke or tumour) and the spinal cord (by an expanded cavity or syrinx), as they emerge in the first thoracic nerve root (by tumour of the apical lung) and as they ascend in the sympathetic plexus around the carotid arteries (by swelling of the arteries in a migrainous attack).

Autonomic nervous system

Structure	Sympathetic effect	Parasympathetic effect
Iris of eye	Dilates pupil	Constricts pupil
Ciliary muscle of eye	Relaxes	Contracts
Salivary glands	Reduces secretion	Increases secretion
Lacrimal gland	Reduces secretion	Increases secretion
Heart	Increases rate and force of contraction	Decreases rate and force of contraction
Bronchi	Dilates	Constricts
Gastrointestinal tract	Decreases motility	Increases motility
Sweat glands	Increases secretion	
Erector pili muscles	Contracts	

Ventricular system and cerebrospinal fluid

The central nervous system contains an interconnecting series of chambers and channels which are derived from the lumen of the embryonic neural tube. In the spinal cord this is represented by the vestigial and insignificant central canal. Within the brain, however, the enormous growth and distortion of the basic tube-like structure is paralleled by the development of an elaborate system of ventricles (Figs 15.1 and 15.2).

TOPOGRAPHICAL ANATOMY OF THE VENTRICULAR SYSTEM

In passing from the spinal cord to the brain stem, the central canal moves progressively more dorsal until, in the rostral (open) medulla, it opens out into a wide and shallow depression, the **fourth ventricle**, on the dorsal surface of the brain stem beneath the cerebellum. The fourth ventricle is rhomboid or diamond-shaped. On each side, a **lateral recess** extends towards the lateral margin of the brain stem and is in continuity, through a small **lateral aperture** (the **foramen of Luschka**), with the subarachnoid space of the

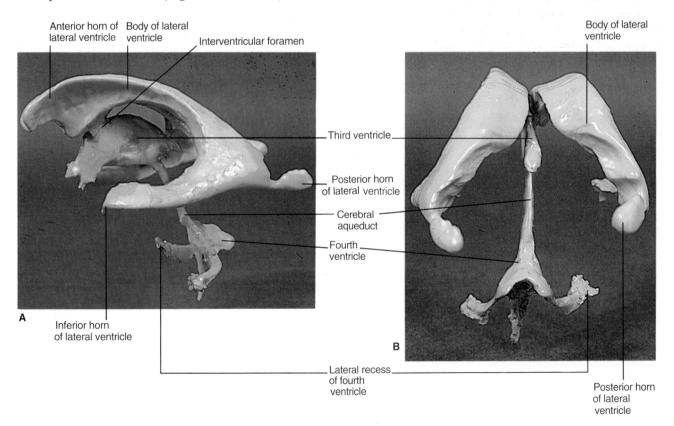

Anterior horn of lateral ventricle · Body of lateral ventricle · Interventricular foramen

Body of lateral ventricle

Third ventricle

Posterior horn of lateral ventricle

Cerebral aqueduct

Fourth ventricle

A

Inferior horn of lateral ventricle

B

Lateral recess of fourth ventricle

Posterior horn of lateral ventricle

Fig. 15.1 **Resin cast of the ventricular system**.
(**A**) Lateral view; (**B**) posterior view.

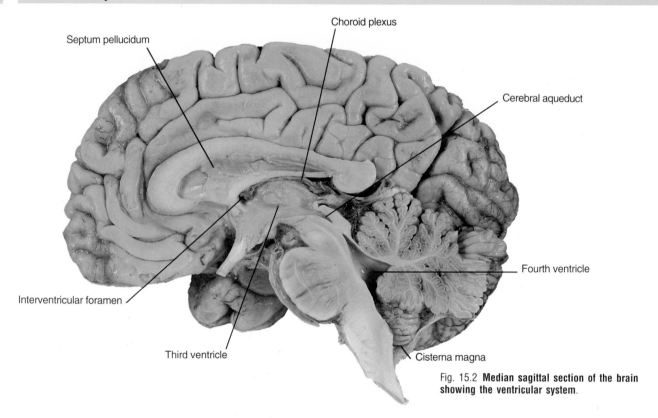

Septum pellucidum

Choroid plexus

Cerebral aqueduct

Fourth ventricle

Interventricular foramen

Third ventricle

Cisterna magna

Fig. 15.2 **Median sagittal section of the brain showing the ventricular system**.

Pons   Basilar artery   Choroid plexus   Facial nerve

Medulla   Olive   Cerebellum

cerebellopontine angle (Fig. 15.3). The roof of the rostral part of the fourth ventricle is partly formed by the superior cerebellar peduncles on either side, the space between them being bridged by the thin superior medullary velum. The caudal part of the roof consists of pia and ependyma, a central defect in which constitutes the **median aperture** of the fourth ventricle, or the **foramen of Magendie**, which provides communication with the cisterna magna (Fig. 15.4).

The fourth ventricle extends rostrally as far as the pontomesencephalic junction where it becomes continuous with the **cerebral aqueduct** which passes throughout the length of the midbrain, beneath the colliculi. At the rostral margin of the midbrain the cerebral aqueduct opens into the **third ventricle** which is a narrow slit-like cavity whose lateral walls are formed by the thalamus and hypothalamus on either side (Figs 9.2 and 15.2). The roof of the ventricle is formed by pia-ependyma which spans between the two striae medullaris thalami, situated along the dorsomedial border of the thalamus. In the rostral part of the third ventricle lies an aperture, the **interventricular foramen**, or **foramen of Monro**, which is located between the column of the fornix and the anterior pole of the thalamus.

Fig. 15.3 **Cerebellopontine angle**.
The point of continuity between the lateral recess of the fourth ventricle and the subarachnoid space is indicated by a small tuft of choroid plexus which protrudes through the lateral aperture.

Superior vermis
of cerebellum

Fig. 15.4 **Posterior view of the brain.** The cerebellum and brain stem have been slightly separated, to show the median aperture of the fourth ventricle.

Median aperture of
fourth ventricle

Dorsal aspect
of medulla

Cerebellar
hemisphere

The interventricular foramen provides communication, on either side, with the extensive **lateral ventricle** located within the cerebral hemisphere (Fig. 13.9). The lateral ventricle is approximately C-shaped. It is usually regarded as consisting of an anterior (frontal) horn, body, posterior (occipital) and inferior (temporal) horns. The **anterior horn** of the lateral ventricle is that part anterior to the interventricular foramen. Its lateral wall is the head of the caudate nucleus and its roof the corpus callosum (Figs 10.4–10.7). The medial wall is formed by the **septum pellucidum**. This thin sheet spans between the corpus callosum and fornix in the midline and separates the anterior horns of the two lateral ventricles. The body of the lateral ventricle extends behind the interventricular foramen, having as its floor the thalamus and tail of the caudate nucleus. More posteriorly the small **posterior horn** extends towards the occipital pole but the principal course of the ventricle sweeps downwards and forwards to form the extensive **inferior horn** which lies in the temporal lobe. In the floor of the inferior horn lies the hippocampus whilst in its roof runs the much attenuated tail of the caudate nucleus (Figs 10.9–10.12).

CEREBROSPINAL FLUID

The ventricular system, together with the cranial and spinal subarachnoid spaces, contains cerebrospinal fluid (CSF). Cerebrospinal fluid is produced by the **choroid plexus** which is located in the lateral, third and fourth ventricles (Figs 13.9 and 15.2). The choroid plexus is

Topographical anatomy

- The ventricular system consists of lateral, third and fourth ventricles and the cerebral aqueduct.
- The lateral ventricle is located within the cerebral hemisphere and is approximately C-shaped. It communicates, via the interventricular foramen, with the third ventricle.
- The third ventricle is a midline, slit-like cavity. Its lateral walls consist of the thalamus and hypothalamus. Caudally, the third ventricle becomes continuous with the cerebral aqueduct.
- The cerebral aqueduct extends throughout the midbrain, linking the third and fourth ventricles.
- The fourth ventricle is located between the brain stem (pons and medulla) and the cerebellum. A median aperture and two lateral apertures communicate with the subarachnoid space surrounding the brain.

formed by invagination of the vascular pia mater into the ventricular lumen, where it becomes highly convoluted, producing a sponge-like appearance. The choroid plexus enters the third and fourth ventricles through their roofs and the lateral ventricle through the choroid fissure, along the line of the fimbria\fornix (Fig. 13.9).

Cerebrospinal fluid is produced partly by an active secretory process and partly by passive diffusion. CSF is a colourless fluid containing little protein and few cells. The volume of CSF in the combined ventricular and

Fig. 15.5 **The cerebral ventricular system and its relationship with the subarachnoid space**. The circulation of cerebrospinal fluid is indicated by arrows.

subarachnoid spaces is of the order of 150 ml. CSF is produced continuously, at a rate sufficient to fill these spaces several times each day. This means that an efficient mechanism is required for the circulation of cerebrospinal fluid and its reabsorption (Fig. 15.5).

Most cerebrospinal fluid is produced by the choroid plexus of the lateral ventricle. From here it flows through the interventricular foramen into the third ventricle and thence, by way of the cerebral aqueduct, into the fourth ventricle. CSF leaves the ventricular system through the three apertures of the fourth ventricle and, thus, enters the subarachnoid space. The majority passes through the median aperture to enter the cisterna magna, located between the medulla and cerebellum. Lesser amounts flow through the lateral apertures to enter the sub-arachnoid space in the region of the cerebellopontine angle. From these sites the majority of CSF flows superiorly, round the cerebral hemispheres, to the sites of reabsorption. Within the subarachnoid space, cerebrospinal fluid serves partially to cushion the brain from sudden movements of the head.

Cerebrospinal fluid is reabsorbed into the venous system by passing into the dural venous sinuses, prin-cipally the superior sagittal sinus. Along the sinuses are located numerous **arachnoid villi** which consist of invaginations of arachnoid mater through the dural wall and into the lumen of the sinus (Fig. 15.6).

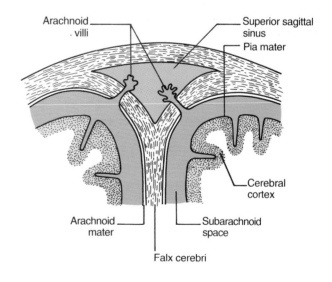

Fig. 15.6 **Transverse section through the superior sagittal sinus showing arachnoid villi**.

Reabsorption occurs at these sites because of the higher hydrostatic pressure in the subarachnoid space than the sinus lumen and because of the greater colloid osmotic pressure of venous blood than CSF. With age the arachnoid villi hypertrophy to form **arachnoid granulations** (Fig. 15.7).

Great longitudinal
fissure

Arachnoid
granulations

Fig. 15.7 **Superior aspect of the cerebral hemispheres showing arachnoid granulations**.

Hydrocephalus

Obstruction of the flow of cerebrospinal fluid within the ventricular system (e.g. by tumours) or the subarachnoid space (e.g. by adhesions following head injury or meningitis) leads to a rise in fluid pressure causing swelling of the ventricles (**hydrocephalus**). The clinical effects are similar to those of a brain tumour and consist of headaches, unsteadiness and mental impairment. Swelling of the optic discs (**papilloedema**) is seen on ophthalmoscopy. Decompression of the dilated ventricles is achieved by inserting a shunt connecting the ventricles to the jugular vein or the abdominal peritoneum.

Cerebrospinal fluid

- Each ventricle contains choroid plexus which secretes cerebrospinal fluid.
- Cerebrospinal fluid flows in the direction: lateral ventricle
  - third ventricle
  - cerebral aqueduct
  - fourth ventricle
  - subarachnoid space.
- The combined ventricular system and subarachnoid space contains about 150 ml of cerebrospinal fluid, this volume being produced several times each day.
- Cerebrospinal fluid is reabsorbed into the venous system through arachnoid villi which project into the superior sagittal dural sinus.

Blood supply of the central nervous system

BLOOD SUPPLY OF THE SPINAL CORD

ARTERIAL SUPPLY OF THE SPINAL CORD
(Fig. 16.1)

Three longitudinal vessels run the length of the spinal cord. These are the single **anterior spinal artery** and the paired **posterior spinal arteries**. The anterior spinal artery arises in a Y-shaped configuration from the two vertebral arteries at the level of the medulla (Fig. 16.2) and descends along the ventral surface of the cord in the midline. The posterior spinal arteries arise from either the vertebral arteries or posterior inferior cerebellar arteries and run caudally on the posterolateral surface of the cord.

The anterior and posterior spinal arteries alone are insufficient to supply the cord below cervical levels and, thus, they receive serial reinforcement by anastomosis

Fig. 16.1 **Schematic drawing of the arterial supply** (red) **and venous drainage** (blue) **of the spinal cord**.
(Modified with permission from Carpenter MB, Sutin J 1983 *Human Neuroanatomy*, 8th edn. Williams and Wilkins, Baltimore.)

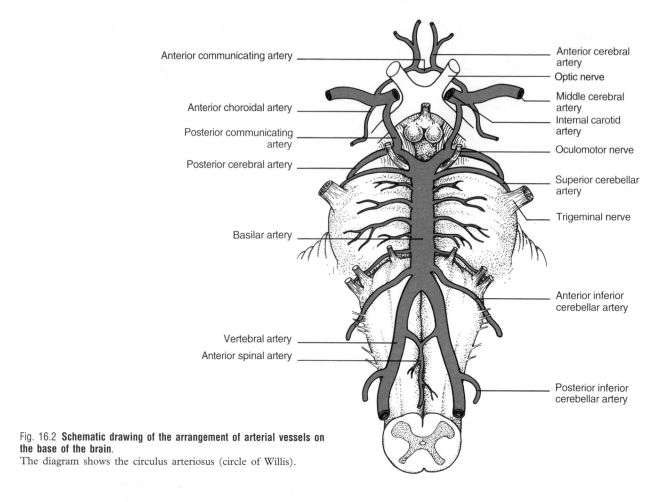

Fig. 16.2 **Schematic drawing of the arrangement of arterial vessels on the base of the brain**.
The diagram shows the circulus arteriosus (circle of Willis).

with **radicular arteries** derived from segmental vessels, including the ascending cervical, intercostal and lumbar arteries. Radicular arteries pass through the intervertebral foramina and divide into anterior and posterior branches which run with the dorsal and ventral spinal nerve roots, respectively. One particularly large radicular artery (the **great radicular artery**, or **artery of Adamkiewicz**) may arise from a lateral intercostal or lumbar artery at any level from T8–L3.

> ### Disorders of blood supply of the spinal cord
>
> The spinal cord and its blood supply are most vulnerable in the thoracic segment and in the anterior portion of the cord. **Occlusion of the anterior spinal artery** leads to an acute thoracic cord syndrome with paraplegia and incontinence. The spinothalamic modalities of pain and temperature are preferentially lost, whereas the proprioceptive functions of the dorsal columns are relatively preserved.

VENOUS DRAINAGE OF THE SPINAL CORD

The venous drainage of the cord follows a basically similar pattern to the arterial supply (Fig. 16.1). Six longitu-

dinal interconnecting venous channels exist. These consist primarily of **anterior** and **posterior spinal veins** which run in the midline. More irregular, sometimes incomplete, bilaterally paired **anterolateral** and **posterolateral veins** are situated near the lines of attachment of the dorsal and ventral nerve roots. All of these vessels drain via **anterior** and **posterior radicular veins** into the **internal vertebral venous plexus** (epidural venous plexus) which is situated between the dura mater and the vertebral periosteum. The internal venous plexus communicates with an **external vertebral venous plexus** and hence with the ascending lumbar veins, the azygos and hemiazygos veins.

> ### Blood supply of the spinal cord
>
> - The spinal cord is supplied by the anterior and posterior spinal arteries, supplemented by radicular arteries.
> - Venous drainage is by anterior and posterior spinal veins which drain, via radicular veins, into the internal vertebral venous plexus.

BLOOD SUPPLY OF THE BRAIN

ARTERIAL SUPPLY OF THE BRAIN
(Figs 16.2–16.6)

The brain is supplied with blood by two pairs of vessels, the internal carotid arteries and the vertebral arteries. The **internal carotid artery** arises from the common carotid artery and enters the middle fossa of the cranial cavity through the carotid canal. Its course then follows a series of characteristic bends, known as the **carotid syphon** (Fig. 16.5), after which it passes forwards through the cavernous sinus, and then upwards on the medial aspect of the anterior clinoid process, reaching the surface of the brain lateral to the optic chiasm. Along its course the internal carotid artery gives rise to a number of preterminal branches:

- **Hypophyseal arteries** arise from the intracavernous section of the internal carotid to supply the neurohypophysis. They also form the pituitary portal system of vessels by which hypothalamic releasing factors are carried to the adenohypophysis.
- The **ophthalmic artery** passes into the orbit through the optic foramen. It supplies the structures of the orbit, the frontal and ethmoidal sinuses, the frontal part of the scalp and dorsum of the nose.

Fig. 16.3 **Arteries on the base of the brain**.
The arterial system has been injected with a red dye.

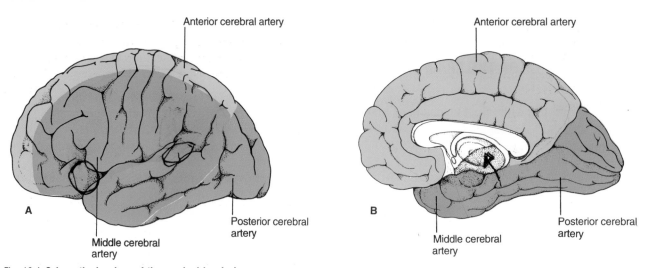

Fig. 16.4 **Schematic drawings of the cerebral hemisphere**.
The diagram shows the cortical distribution of the three cerebral arteries. (**A**) Lateral aspect; (**B**) medial aspect.

- The **anterior choroidal artery** supplies the optic tract, the choroid plexus of the lateral ventricle, the hippocampus and some of the deep structures of the hemisphere, including the internal capsule and globus pallidus.
- The **posterior communicating artery** passes backwards to join the posterior cerebral artery, thus forming part of the circle of Willis.

Lateral to the optic chiasma, the internal carotid artery divides into its two terminal branches, the **anter**ior and **middle cerebral arteries**. The anterior cerebral artery courses medially above the optic nerve and then passes into the great longitudinal fissure between the frontal lobes. As it does so, it is joined to the corresponding vessel of the opposite side by the short **anterior communicating artery**. Within the great longitudinal fissure, the anterior cerebral artery follows the dorsal curvature of the corpus callosum, branches ramifying over the medial surface of the frontal and parietal lobes, which it supplies (Fig. 16.4). The territory supplied by the anterior cerebral artery, therefore,

Fig. 16.5 **Carotid angiograms**.
Radio-opaque material has been introduced into the internal carotid artery in order to display its intracranial course and distribution. (**A**) Lateral view; (**B**) antero-posterior (Towne's) view. (Courtesy of Dr. P. Griffiths, Department of Radiology, Newcastle General Hospital, Newcastle-upon-Tyne.)

includes the motor and sensory cortices for the lower limb. Fine terminal branches also extend out of the great longitudinal fissure to supply a narrow lateral band of frontal and parietal cortices.

The middle cerebral artery is the largest of the three cerebral arteries and its cortical territory is the largest (Fig. 16.4). It passes laterally from its origin to enter the lateral fissure within which it subdivides, branches supplying virtually the whole of the lateral surface of the frontal, parietal and temporal lobes. This includes the primary motor and sensory cortices for the whole of the body, excluding the lower limb. It also serves the auditory cortex and the insula within the depths of the lateral fissure.

Since the structures supplied by branches of the internal carotid artery are normally perfused almost entirely from this source, they are often referred to as being supplied by the 'internal carotid system'.

The **vertebral artery** arises from the subclavian artery, ascends through the foramina transversaria of the cervical vertebrae and enters the cranial cavity through the foramen magnum, alongside the ventrolateral aspect of the medulla (Figs 16.2, 16.3 and 16.6). As they pass rostrally, the two vertebral arteries converge, uniting at the junction between medulla and pons to form the midline **basilar artery**. Along its course the vertebral artery gives rise to a number of branches, including the anterior and posterior spinal arteries which supply the medulla and spinal cord. Its largest branch

is the **posterior inferior cerebellar artery** which supplies the inferior aspect of the cerebellum.

The basilar artery runs the length of the pons, which it supplies by means of many small pontine branches. It also gives rise to the **anterior inferior cerebellar artery**, which supplies the anterior and inferior portion of the cerebellum, and the **labyrinthine artery**, which passes into the internal acoustic meatus to supply the inner ear. At the junction of the pons and midbrain the basilar artery divides into two pairs of vessels, the **superior cerebellar arteries** and the **posterior cerebral arteries**. The superior cerebellar artery supplies the superior aspect of the cerebellum. The posterior cerebral artery curves around the midbrain to supply the visual cortex of the occipital lobe and the inferomedial aspect of the temporal lobe (Fig. 16.4).

The brain regions (brain stem, cerebellum and occipital lobe) served by the vertebral and basilar arteries and their branches are described as being supplied by the 'vertebrobasilar system'.

The internal carotid and vertebrobasilar systems are joined by two thin vessels, the **posterior communicating arteries**, which pass rostrocaudally between the end of the internal carotid and the posterior cerebral arteries. This completes an anastomosis of vessels on the base of the brain, known as the **circulus arteriosus** or **circle of Willis** (Figs 16.2 and 16.3), which encircles the optic chiasma and the floor of the hypothalamus

Fig. 16.6 **Vertebral angiograms.**
Radio-opaque material has been introduced into the vertebral artery in order to display its intracranial course and distribution.
(**A**) Lateral view; (**B**) antero-posterior (Towne's) view. (Courtesy of Dr. P. Griffiths, Department of Radiology, Newcastle General Hospital, Newcastle-upon-Tyne.)

Disorders of blood supply of the brain

One of the commonest causes of neurological disability is **stroke**. The sudden occlusion of a cerebral artery leads to death of brain tissue (**infarction**). Rupture of a blood vessel causes bleeding into the brain (**cerebral haemorrhage**). These events lead to the rapid development of a focal neurological syndrome. Strokes related to the carotid artery and its cerebral branches are associated with focal epilepsy, a contralateral sensory/motor deficit and a psychological deficit (e.g. aphasia). Strokes involving the vertebrobasilar circulation lead to a focal brain stem syndrome. Recovery of function can occur but may take up to two years and can be incomplete.

An **aneurysm** is an abnormal, balloon-like, swelling of an artery. A surgical emergency arises when an aneurysm ruptures and blood projects around the brain in the subarachnoid space (**subarachnoid haemorrhage**) and into the brain (**intracerebral haemorrhage**). A sudden severe headache and neck stiffness are followed by coma and neurological deficits. Neurosurgery is required to seal the aneurysm to prevent further bleeding and allow recovery.

An **angioma**, or **arteriovenous malformation**, is a congenital collection of swollen blood vesels which can rupture, causing cerebral haemorrhage, or 'steal' blood from adjacent brain regions leading to epilepsy and a focal cerebral syndrome.

Arterial supply of the brain

- The brain is supplied by paired internal carotid and vertebral arteries.
- The internal carotid artery terminates lateral to the optic chiasma, giving rise to the anterior and middle cerebral arteries.
- The anterior cerebral artery passes into the great longitudinal fissure and supplies the medial aspect of the cerebral hemisphere.
- The middle cerebral artery passes into the lateral fissure and supplies the lateral aspect of the cerebral hemisphere.
- The vertebral arteries run on the ventrolateral aspect of the medulla, uniting to form the midline basilar artery which extends the length of the pons. Along their course the vertebral and basilar arteries give rise to branches which supply the cerebellum and brain stem.
- The principal terminal branch of the basilar artery is the posterior cerebral artery which supplies the occipital lobe of the cerebral hemisphere.
- The anterior communicating artery links together the two anterior cerebral arteries. Posterior communicating arteries pass between the internal carotid artery and posterior cerebral artery, on each side. This anastomosis of vessels constitutes the circle of Willis.
- Small perforating arteries arise from the circle of Willis to supply the hypothalamic area and the internal capsule.

and midbrain. The anastomotic arrangement of vessels provides the possibility that obstruction or narrowing of the proximal parts of the cerebral arteries, which would be expected to lead to insufficiency in the perfusion of their territories, might be compensated by circulation of blood through the communicating arteries. The actual significance of this arrangement is dependent upon the size of the communicating arteries, which is highly variable between individuals. From the arteries which constitute the circle of Willis, numerous small vessels penetrate the surface of the brain. These are known as the **perforating arteries** (central or ganglionic arteries) and are considered to consist of two groups.

- **Anterior perforating arteries** arise from the anterior cerebral artery, anterior communicating artery and the region of origin of the middle cerebral artery. They enter the brain in the region between the optic chiasma and the termination of the olfactory tract, known as the anterior perforated substance. These vessels supply large parts of the basal ganglia, the optic chiasma, the internal capsule and hypothalamus.
- The **posterior perforating arteries** arise from the posterior cerebral and posterior communicating arteries. They enter the brain in the region between the two crura cerebri of the midbrain, known as the posterior perforated substance, to supply the ventral portion of the midbrain and parts of the subthalamus and hypothalamus.

VENOUS DRAINAGE OF THE BRAIN

Three sets of vessels take part in venous drainage of the brain (Figs 16.7 and 16.8): the superficial veins, the deep veins and the dural venous sinuses. None of these vessels contain valves. **Superficial veins** lie within the subarachnoid space (Fig. 16.7). **Superior cerebral veins** primarily drain the lateral surface of the cerebral hemispheres and empty into the superior sagittal sinus. The **superficial middle cerebral vein** runs along the line of the lateral fissure and empties into the cavernous sinus. In addition, two major anastomotic channels exist, the superior (great) anastomotic vein and the inferior anastomotic vein, which drain into the superior sagittal sinus and the transverse sinus, respectively.

Deep cerebral veins drain the internal structures of the forebrain. Of particular note are the **thalamostriate vein** and the **choroidal vein** which drain the basal ganglia, thalamus, internal capsule, choroid plexus and hippocampus. These vessels merge to form

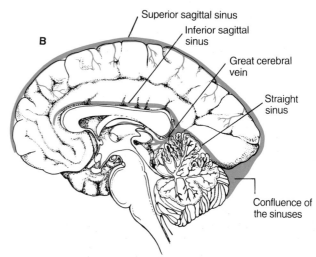

Fig. 16.7 **Venous drainage of the brain**.
(**A**) Lateral view; (**B**) sagittal view.

the **internal cerebral vein**. The two internal cerebral veins then unite in the midline to form the **great cerebral vein** (of Galen), which lies beneath the splenium of the corpus callosum. This short vessel is continuous with the straight sinus which lies in the midline of the tentorium cerebelli.

The cerebral veins drain into the **dural venous sinuses** (Figs 16.7 and 16.8; see also Ch. 4) which are channels formed between the two layers of dura mater. Major venous sinuses are located in the attached borders of the falx cerebri and the tentorium cerebelli and on the floor of the cranial cavity.

Along the line where the falx cerebri attaches to the interior of the cranium lies the **superior sagittal sinus**. This receives blood primarily from the superior cerebral veins which ramify over the lateral surface of the cerebral hemispheres. The free border of the falx encloses the smaller **inferior sagittal sinus** into which flow veins on the medial aspect of the hemisphere. Within the tentorium cerebelli, along the line of its attachment to the falx, lies the large **straight sinus**. Into this runs the great cerebral vein, which drains the deep structures of the forebrain, and also the inferior sagittal sinus.

The superior sagittal sinus and the straight sinus converge at the **confluence of the sinuses** which lies adjacent to the internal occipital protuberance. From here, blood flows laterally on either side in the **transverse sinus** which lies along the line of attachment of the tentorium to the occipital bone. The transverse sinus is continuous with the **sigmoid sinus** which in turn joins the **internal jugular vein** at the level of the jugular foramen.

The **cavernous sinus** (Fig. 16.8) lies lateral to the body of the sphenoid bone. It receives blood from the

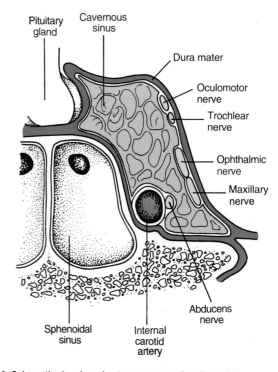

Fig. 16.8 **Schematic drawing of a transverse section through the cavernous sinus**.

Diseases of the venous sinuses

Thrombosis of the sagittal sinuses is a rare complication of childbirth, blood clotting disorders and ear infection. Obstruction of the venous drainage of the brain leads to cerebral swelling (**oedema**) and the syndrome of **raised intracranial pressure** (p. 32). Cerebral damage due to venous infarction manifests as epileptic seizures and focal paralysis of the limbs.

middle cerebral vein and drains into the internal jugular vein (via the inferior petrosal sinus) and into the transverse sinus (via the superior petrosal sinus). The two cavernous sinuses are connected by intercavernous sinuses which lie anterior and posterior to the hypophysis forming a venous circle around it (the circular sinus). The dural venous sinuses are connected to extracranial veins via **emissary veins**.

Venous drainage of the brain

- Venous drainage of the brain involves superficial veins, deep veins and dural venous sinuses.
- Superficial veins empty principally into the superior sagittal sinus and the cavernous sinus.
- Deep cerebral veins drain into the great cerebral vein which is continuous with the straight sinus.
- The superior sagittal sinus and straight sinuses meet at the confluence of the sinuses.
- Venous blood flows, via the transverse sinus and sigmoid sinus, into the internal jugular vein.

Glossary

Acalculia: Inability to calculate.

Accommodation: Act of refocussing the visual image.

Acromegaly: Overgrowth of the skeleton and organs due to excessive release of growth hormone from a pituitary tumour.

Acuity: Resolving power.

Adenoma: Benign tumour.

Adhesion: Scarring of tissues, fixing them together.

Adipsia: Inability, or loss of desire, to drink.

Aetiology: Relating to the cause of disease.

Afferent: Carrying towards (e.g. cerebellar afferent neurones carry impulses to the cerebellum).

Agnosia: Inability to recognise objects.

Agraphia: Inability to write.

Akinesia: Loss, or slowness, of movement.

Alexia: Inability to read.

Amnesia: Loss of memory.

Anastomosis: Intercommunication between vessels (e.g. circulus arteriosus or Circle of Willis).

Aneurysm: Abnormal dilatation of an artery.

Angioma: Congenital swollen collection of blood vessels.

Anomia: Inability to name objects.

Antidiuretic: An agent which reduces the volume of urine produced by the kidney.

Aphagia: Inability, or loss of desire, to eat.

Aphasia: Loss of ability to use language.

Apraxia: Loss of skilled movements despite preservation of power, sensation and coordination.

Areflexia: Loss of reflexes.

Ataxia: Loss of ability to coordinate voluntary movements.

Atrophy: Wasting or degeneration.

Baroreceptor: Neuronal sensory ending which detects changes in arterial blood pressure.

Biopsy: Tissue sample taken from a patient for the diagnosis of disease.

Bulimia: Overeating disorder.

Bradykinesia: Slowness of movement.

Bulbar palsy: Weakness of tongue, pharynx and larynx due to disease of the lower cranial nerves.

Cataract: Opacity of the lens of the eye, leading to deterioration of vision.

Cephalic: Relating to the head.

Chemoreceptor: Neuronal sensory ending which detects changes in the chemical composition of circulating blood.

Chiasma: Decussation or crossing over of nerve fibres (e.g. optic chiasma).

Chorea: Involuntary, jerky movements of the face and limbs.

Coma: Prolonged and unnatural state of unconsciousness.

Computed tomography (CT): Imaging technique utilising X-rays to visualise the structure of the nervous system.

Concussion: Loss of consciousness due to head injury.

Contralateral: Relating to the opposite side.

Contusion: Bruising.

Convulsion: Involuntary contraction or spasm of muscles.

Cordotomy: Neurosurgical procedure to destroy specific pathways in the spinal cord.

Craniopharyngioma: Congenital tumour of the base of the brain.

Craniotomy: Neurosurgical procedure to open the cranial cavity.

Cushing's disease: Overgrowth of the adrenal glands causing excessive release of corticosteroid hormones.

Decussation: Crossing over of nerve fibres from one side of the central nervous system to the other (e.g. pyramidal decussation).

Dementia: Loss of mental abilities.

Demyelination: Loss of the myelin sheath surrounding neuronal axons.

Diabetes insipidus: Failure of the posterior pituitary gland causing reduced release of antidiuretic hormone.

Dysarthria: Inability to pronounce.

Dysphagia: Inability to swallow.

Dysphonia: Inability to produce the voice.

Efferent: Carrying away from (e.g. striatal efferent fibres carry impulses away from the striatum).

Electroencephalography (EEG): Technique to detect the surface electrical activity of the brain.

Electromyography: Technique to determine the electrical activity of muscles.

Emetic: Causing nausea and vomiting.

Encephalopathy: Disorder of the brain.

Epilepsy: Paroxysmal attack of disturbed consciousness and sensorimotor function due to abnormal electrophysiological discharges of the brain.

Fasciculation: Spontaneous contraction of denervated motor units, visible on inspection.

Fasciculus: Bundle of nerve fibres (e.g. medial longitudinal fasciculus).

Febrile: Refers to raised body temperature (fever).

Fibrillation: Spontaneous contraction of denervated muscle fibres, detected on electromyography (EMG).

Foramen: An opening (e.g. foramen magnum).

Ganglion: A collection of nerve cell bodies outside the CNS (e.g. dorsal root ganglion).

General paralysis of the insane (GPI): Disease of the frontal lobes due to late neurosyphilis.

Glioma: Tumour derived from glial cells.

Haematoma: Blood clot.

Hallucination: Abnormal perceptual experience.

Hemianopia: Loss of sight affecting one half of the visual field (e.g. bitemporal hemianopia).

Hemiparesis: Weakness of one side of the body.

Hepatolenticular degeneration (Wilson's disease): Inherited disease of copper metabolism affecting the liver and brain.

Herpes zoster: Virus causing shingles (q.v.).

Huntington's disease: Inherited degenerative disease of the brain causing chorea (q.v.) and dementia (q.v.).

Hyperacusis: Increased hearing sensitivity.

Hyperreflexia: Abnormal increase in reflex activity.

Hypertonia: Abnormal increase in muscle tone.

Hypertrophy: Enlargement of tissues.

Hypothyroidism: Underactivity of the thyroid gland causing reduced release of thyroid hormone.

Hypotonia: Abnormal decrease in muscle tone.

Idiopathic: Of unknown cause.

Infarction: Death of tissue due to impairment of its circulation.

Ipsilateral: Relating to the same side.

Kinaesthesia: Perception of movement.

Lamina: A thin layer (e.g. internal medullary lamina).

Lesion: Site of disease or damage.

Lobectomy: Surgical resection of lobe of the brain.

Lumen: A space or cavity.

Lymphoma: Tumour of the lymphoid system.

Magnetic resonance imaging (MRI): Technique to image the structure of the nervous system, which does not employ ionising radiation.

Mastication: The act of chewing.

Miosis: Pupillary constriction.

Meningitis: Inflammation of the meninges.

Metastasis: Spread of tumour to distant sites.

Migraine: Paroxysmal headache.

Motor neurone disease: Degenerative disease of upper and lower motor neurones, causing paralysis.

Multiple sclerosis: Immune disease of the central nervous system, causing relapsing disorder of nervous function.

Muscular dystrophy: Inherited degeneration of muscles, causing progressive paralysis.

Myasthenia gravis: Immune disorder of the neuromuscular junction, causing muscular fatigue.

Myopathy: Disease of muscle.

Narcolepsy: Paroxysmal sleep attacks.

Necrosis: Death of tissue.

Neoplasia: Tumorous overgrowth of tissue.

Neurofibromatosis: Inherited disease causing tumours of meninges, central nervous system, peripheral nerves and skin.

Neuroma: Tumour derived from nerve cells.

Neuropathy: Disease of nerve cells.

Neurosyphilis: Infection of the nervous system due to spirochaete.

Nociception: Sensitivity to noxious stimuli.

Nucleus: Structure within a cell which contains chromosomal DNA; also a collection of nerve cell bodies within the CNS (e.g. dentate nucleus).

Nystagmus: To and fro movements of the eyes.

Oedema: Swelling due to accumulated fluid.

Oligodendroglioma: Tumour derived from oligodendroglia.

Ophthalmoscopy: Clinical examination of the eye with an ophthalmoscope.

Palsy: Weakness.

Papilloedema: Swelling of the optic nerve(s).

Paraesthesia: Tingling sensations ('pins and needles').

Paraphasia: Use of incorrect word.

Paraplegia: Weakness or paralysis of the legs.

Paresis: Muscular weakness.

Parkinson's disease: Disease of the basal ganglia causing akinesia (q.v.), rigidity (q.v.) and tremor (q.v.).

Paroxysm: Sudden attack.

Photophobia: Intolerance to light.

Plexus: Structure consisting of interwoven nerves (e.g. brachial plexus) or blood vessels (e.g. choroid plexus).

Poliomyelitis: Viral infection of motor neurones of the spinal cord and brain stem.

Positron emission tomography (PET): technique for imaging the function of the brain.

Prolapse: Displacement from normal anatomical position.

Proprioception: The detection of position and movement of body parts.

Pseudobulbar palsy: Weakness of the tongue, pharynx and larynx due to disease of the corticobulbar tracts.

Psychosis: Abnormal mental state with altered precepts (hallucinations) and false ideas (delusions).

Ptosis: Abnormal drooping of the eyelid.

Quadriplegia: Paralysis affecting all four limbs.

Rheumatic fever: Immune disease of the joints, heart and brain following bacterial infection.

Rigidity: Increased resistance to passive movement of the limbs throughout their range.

Schizophrenia: Disease of the brain causing psychosis (q.v.).

Seizure: Sudden disturbance of consciousness or sensorimotor function.

Shingles: Infection of the ganglia of cranial and spinal nerves by herpes zoster virus (q.v.).

Single photon emission tomography (SPECT): Technique for imaging the function of the brain.

Somatic: Relating to body parts other than the viscera.

Somatotopic: The orderly representation of body parts in the CNS.

Spasticity: Increased resistance to passive movement of the limbs when muscles are initially stretched.

Spondylosis: Degeneration of the spine.

Stroke: Sudden neurological deficit due to disease of the circulation to the brain.

Sydenham's chorea: Manifestation of rheumatic fever (q.v.) affecting the basal ganglia and causing involuntary movements.

Syncope: Fainting attack.

Syndrome: Group of signs and symptoms which characterise a disease.

Syringobulbia: Expanding cavity (syrinx) within the medulla.

Syringomyelia: Expanding cavity within the spinal cord.

Thalamotomy: Neurosurgical destruction of part of the thalamus.

Thrombosis: Coagulation of blood in artery or vein.

Tract: An aggregation of nerve cell processes having more or less the same origin and destination (e.g. corticospinal tract).

Tremor: Trembling of head or limbs.

Index